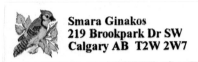
Smara Ginakos
219 Brookpark Dr SW
Calgary AB T2W 2W7

THE ESSENCE OF BEAUTY

Adrianna Scheibner, M.D.

THE ESSENCE OF BEAUTY

An indispensable guide to living in health and beauty for people who care about the quality of life.

Adrianna Scheibner, M.D.

A & A Publishers & Distributors, Los Angeles

THE ESSENCE OF BEAUTY

Library of Congress Catalog Card Number 93-71597.

ISBN 0-9636481-0-1

Published by A & A Publishers and Distributors, Inc.

Typeset by Bonnie Fox & Associates.

Photographs of author by Eddie Garcia.

Printed in the United States of America by Arcata Graphics.

To my son, Aaron, whose compassion, wisdom and patience are a daily inspiration to me.

ACKNOWLEDGEMENTS

I wish to express my eternal gratitude to Professor Gerald Milton and Professor William McCarthy for introducing me to the world of lasers and skin cancer research and for their confidence in my abilities, their encouragement and support. I would also like to extend special thanks to Arnold Klein, M.D.; Harry Glassman, M.D.; Kenneth Arndt, M.D.; Ronald Wheeland, M.D.; John Yarborough, M.D.; Rox Anderson, M.D.; Lesley Wild, M.D.; Peter Muzikants, M.D.; Neal Hamilton, M.D.; Annie Millar and Peter Azer for their unequivocal support of my work over the last several years through their own dedication of excellence; which made not only this book possible, but my most recent contributions to laser dermatology. A heartfelt thanks to Rox Anderson, M.D., of Harvard Medical School for conceiving and developing the pulsed dye laser and to Horace Furumoto and Shaun Cave and their team at Cynosure Corporation for the development and refinement of the medical pulsed dye laser which has made it possible for me to develop techniques for the laser treatment of scars.

Among the many other people to whom I am thankful for their advice, expertise and contribution in putting together this book, I offer my particular thanks to: David Duffy, M.D.; Dennis Thompson, M.D.; N. Milstein, M.D.; the Collagen Corporation; the Dow Corning Corporation; the FDA for providing information; and Kodak for the superior quality of their film. To Suze Curtis, Owen Meldy, Lee and Darrien Iacocca, and Lucille Ostrow, for their encouraging and helpful comments, and special friendship, and to all the people whose words of wisdom are quoted herein; and, above all to Peter Azer for his invaluable advice, intuition, patience and exceptional support in the writing of this manuscript. I thank Joe Gallagher for his patience and wisdom in editing it; Mark Brammeier for his cartoon illustrations, Colette Kay, David Fruth and Bonnie Fox for their dedication, patience, and especially long hours in accomplishing the final steps in putting this manuscript into the reader's hands.

In addition to the special individuals listed above, I wish to extend my thanks and deep gratitude to all the patients with scars and skin blemishes, who were told nothing could be done about their problem but who inspite of this discouragement still refused to give up and continued to believe that someone, somewhere, would be able to treat them. Thank you for your faith and your prayers.

Finally, I wish to thank my parents for providing me with all the necessary attributes and strength of character that has helped me achieve whatever I have undertaken despite adversity and what at times seemed like a never-ending stream of obstacles to be worked into opportunities.

DISCLAIMER

The medical procedures described in The Essence Of Beauty, should be performed by qualified professionals. As pointed out in the text, the results vary from person to person and cannot be predicted with accuracy and certainly not guaranteed to have a certain outcome. No responsibility can be taken for the work of any professional whose assistance is sought after reading this book.

If you have any questions regarding this material, consult your physician or direct your inquiries to the author at the following address:

436 North Bedford Drive, #205
Beverly Hills, CA 90210

FOREWORD

I first met Dr. Adrianna Scheibner in 1986 when she presented her work at the American Society of Laser Medicine and Surgery. What impressed me most was not only the unsurpassed excellence of her work, but even at that time she had single-handedly treated more patients than all the doctors using lasers to treat skin problems in the entire United States! Needless to say, continuing to treat patients on a full-time basis, Dr. Scheibner has since then successfully treated over 10,000 scars using techniques she developed even more recently. The methods Dr. Scheibner developed in the early eighties had for the first time eliminated the scarring which was so common prior to her break-through contribution. Dr. Scheibner made it possible to treat children and showed what miracles could result from the combination of art and science. It was as a result of seeing what could be done that motivated me to devote my practice to the use of lasers.

What impressed me even more was the compassion with which Dr. Scheibner spoke about her patients. As a pediatric dermatologist, I share this love and compassion for children, big and small. It is amazing what a difference it can make in a child's life to have a treatment which can eliminate a disfiguring skin condition. It is truly life saving.

But, not only children have benefited from these procedures. We sometimes forget that adults are but grown-up versions of children. There are many wonderful procedures now available in dermatology and plastic surgery that can repair or enhance ones appearance and as Dr. Scheibner points out, although external beauty does help people feel better, beauty and happiness are primarily an inside job. It is a matter of learning the most we can about our internal processes of thinking and feeling and what can be done on the physical level that will enhance the quality of life.

In Dr. Scheibner's usual style of excellence, this book accomplishes that goal.

Michael Bond, M.D.
Pediatric Dermatologist
Memphis, Tennessee

TABLE OF CONTENTS

PART ONE
Beauty From Within

PART TWO
External Beauty

INTRODUCTION

The idea for writing this book came as a result of the many questions asked about skin care and appearance-improving procedures by the thousands of patients I have treated since I began performing laser treatments in 1980.

More importantly, beyond the questions and beyond the problems to be treated, whether large or small, I always found a human being looking for the most elusive answer of all: that of self-worth and happiness. I have heard time and again, "If only I had thinner legs...," "If only I didn't have broken capillaries...," "If only I had a smaller nose...I would be happy."

It is true, whether we like it or not, that we live in a world where appearance counts. Beauty makes the first impression, and however much we'd like to think society has changed, beauty is still a source of social power. However, without true self-appreciation, a beautiful appearance is a source of external power only, which at best is temporary and subject to too many unsettling external influences.

To tell you only what you can do physically to enhance your appearance would be to withhold the most valuable information of all: information that can help you achieve happiness regardless of your appearance and enable you to give yourself the most precious gift of all – that of love and appreciation of your true self. This love is the real reason for the quest for external beauty.

You are all beautiful within. I trust *The Essence of Beauty* will help you to see and appreciate it. The first part of this book is about true self-appreciation which comes from within. The second part is to serve as a guide to safe and wise use of simple and not-so-simple procedures used to keep skin looking youthful so that you can look and feel your best at any age.

PART ONE

BEAUTY FROM WITHIN

CHAPTER

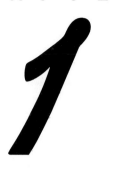

WHY WE DESIRE BEAUTY

THE VALUE OF BEAUTY IN OUR SOCIETY

Looking good seems to have become a preoccupation in our society today. It is undoubtedly true that if we think we look good, we feel good about ourselves.

But why is that so? What is it about thinking we look attractive that makes us feel good?

Is it because the reaction of people to beauty is more positive which, in turn, affects the way we think and feel about ourselves, creating a positive mental attitude in everyone's mind?

> *A positive attitude is crucial for our self-image,*
> *for when we perceive our body in positive terms,*
> *we feel a sense of well-being and love; if we deval-*
> *ue our body, we may feel discomfort and resent-*
> *ment.*
>
> **Rita Freedman**

A positive mental attitude, in fact, determines the quality of our whole life and is most likely the real aim behind the desire to look attractive.

No matter how skillful the surgeon or how incredible the results, if

we do not think we look better after a cosmetic procedure and, therefore, do not feel better about ourselves, then the treatment as far as we
are concerned, has failed.

In other words, it is not physical beauty itself but what **we make of
it through our own thoughts** that really matters.

That our thoughts are crucial in determining the kind and quality of
life we lead, has been known and taught by teachers and philosophers
for thousands of years. As the Greek philosopher Epictetus said two
thousand years ago;

> *People are disturbed not by things, but by the
> view they take of them.*

It is the physician's responsibility to do his or her best. But it is ours
to be happy and to make the best of the results.

"Body-loathing," as defined by Dr. Rita Freedman in her book
Bodylove, results in a "pre-occupation and dissatisfaction with appearance that causes anxiety, guilt, and shame over 'flaws' real and imag-
ined." Body-loathing wounds both the mind and the body and erodes
our sense of self-esteem, thus adversely affecting our daily life.

But where does the injury come from? It is not society or the external pressure that does this to us. It is **what we do to ourselves** as a
result of our own **thinking** that does the harm.

Someone's negative comment can hurt us only if we buy what they
say as being the truth. The closer to truth we believe the comment to
be, the more upset we will become. Thus, if we do not feel good about
ourselves, we will be very sensitive to any remarks pertaining to our
perceived weakness.

Take the following example. Someone says to us, "The sky is never
blue. How foolish thinking that the sky can ever be blue!" In this example it is easy for our response to be detached, and if our sense of
esteem is good we may just laugh at the ridiculousness of the accusa-
tion that we are foolish and wonder which planet the person came
from!

If, however, someone says, "You are not attractive," and we ourselves believe this to be true, we will be cut to the core and feel hurt
and depressed. These unpleasant emotions will last as long as it takes

for our own inner thoughts and feelings of being unattractive to dissipate, be replaced by other positive thoughts or feelings, or just be forgotten.

In other words, no one can hurt us unless we, ourselves, accept the hurtful remark as being a true description of who we are. That is, the problem lies not in other people and what they say and do to us but in our own **reaction** to them.

We can choose our own reaction to any external event, and this ability to take control of ourselves is our true source of self-worth, internal strength, and self-command.

Numerous surveys indicate that over the last two decades women, in particular, have become less and less satisfied with their bodies and themselves. As this volume's bibliography bears out, countless books have been written about acquiring self-acceptance and self-esteem.

This dissatisfaction has serious consequences as the image we have of ourselves, which is created by our own thoughts, is crucial in determining the quality of our whole life.

> *Our self-image prescribes the limits for the accomplishment of any particular goals. It prescribes the **area of the possible**.*
>
> Maxwell Maltz

That is, what we think about ourselves determines not only how we feel but also what we do in life, our happiness and success.

All that really matters is **how we think about ourselves and NOT how we actually look.**

This factual observation is not intended to dissuade you from seeking to look attractive or from obtaining treatment to look younger. The first part of this book is intended to provide you with the keys to **self-knowledge** and **self-acceptance** that will enable you to look at what follows in the second part as describing choices you can make if you wish, not necessities you cannot live without—and to make the best of the treatments once you have chosen to obtain them.

The keys to self-knowledge and self-acceptance consist of understanding how and what we think and the tremendous power and far-reaching influence our thoughts have in creating our feelings, beliefs, attitudes, and our entire destiny and what we can do to enhance our strengths and eliminate our weaknesses.

You could be the most beautiful woman or the most handsome man in the world, but if you don't think so and you continue to think negatively about yourself or some aspect of your life, not only will you limit your potential but you could actually make your negative beliefs come to pass.

I have seen the most tragic consequences of such negative beliefs in women and men who were beautiful or handsome to begin with but did not think they were. Driven by their negative beliefs about their appearance, they underwent one cosmetic procedure after another; eventually they became scarred or distorted in their appearance, which they finally appreciated only after it was lost.

Fortunately, these instances are rare. The great majority of people who have cosmetic procedures do obtain desirable results and do feel better about themselves. The positive thoughts and feelings about their appearance seem to produce more positive thoughts and feelings in other areas of their life. **It is this positivity in thinking** resulting from any cosmetic appearance-improving procedure or treatment, including skin care, **that you are actually buying.**

To be successful, to create and enjoy quality life, we need to feel good about ourselves and to **believe in ourselves with our whole being.** Believe that we can be whatever we want to be; that we can do whatever we set our mind to accomplish, provided, of course, it is beneficial to us and does not cause harm to anyone; and that we are worthwhile, deserving human beings whether or not we accomplish our constructive desires. No one else—no external circumstances or material possessions—can give us belief in ourselves.

BELIEVING IN OURSELVES IS A CHOICE WE MAKE DAY BY DAY, MOMENT BY MOMENT. IT IS A GIFT WE GIVE TO OURSELVES EVERY MOMENT OF OUR LIFE.

Belief in ourselves is the very substance of who we are. It gives us resilience and drive and the ability to overcome any difficulty we may encounter. When we believe in ourselves we can accomplish anything our mind can conceive and believe.

Everything is possible for him who believes.

Mark 9:23

Thus, how we think about ourselves is the very foundation of our life. And so the real reason we want to think and feel we are beautiful is that we want to feel good about ourselves. When we feel good about ourselves, we are more likely to appreciate our full potential. And to achieve it.

C H A P T E R

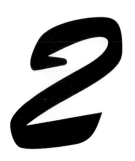

THINKING BEAUTIFUL

HOW WE THINK IS MORE IMPORTANT THAN HOW WE LOOK

You think and your thoughts materialize as experience; and thus it is, all unknown to yourself as a rule, that you are actually weaving the pattern of your own destiny, here and now, by the way in which you allow yourself to think, day by day and all day long. Your fate is largely in your hands. Nobody but yourself can keep you down. Neither parents, nor wives, nor husbands, nor employers, nor neighbors, nor poverty, nor ignorance, nor any power whatever can keep you out of your own when once you have learned how to think.

Emmet Fox

WHAT ARE THOUGHTS?

By definition, the word *thought* refers to any mental activity. To better understand how and why our thoughts have such profound influence on our life, it is first useful to know what happens physiologically when we think.

Thoughts are processed and generated by the physical entity of our brain by means of electrical activity. Although these electrical impulses form an infinite variety of brain wave patterns, researchers have to date identified four types which in a general way indicate what type of thinking the brain is engaged in. These different types of thinking patterns are also associated with certain general types of mental or feeling states.

The four general types of brain wave patterns are:

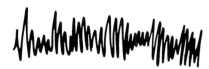

1. Beta waves – These are rapidly occurring brain waves which are predominant during the time we are awake, mentally alert and thinking consciously, concentrating our attention on our environment. They include the self-talk or "monkey chatter" in which we engage most of the time we are awake, whether we are aware of it or not, as well as the conscious positive and negative thoughts. Our moods or the feelings we experience will be positive or negative depending on whether our thoughts in the beta range are positive or negative.

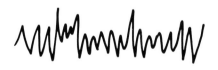

2. Alpha waves – are slower. They are associated with a positive state of relaxation and cessation of the "monkey chatter".

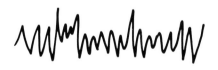

3. Theta waves - are very slow brain waves. They indicate a state of deep reverie, visualization, creative thinking, elation and bliss; all

very positive states of consciousness.

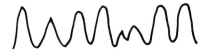

4. Delta waves – are ultra slow and occur only during deep sleep.

In children, up to about age fourteen, theta waves predominate, whereas in adults beta waves are most commonly produced in the "normal" awake state. The predominance of theta waves in childhood could explain the child-like mental state of spontaneous mental imagery and imaginative, creative thinking.

The brain is composed of two halves or hemispheres. The right side of the brain is better able to process what we see, spatial and creative information while the left brain is better able to process verbal tasks such as language skills, mathematics and other rational processes.

When brain waves are measured simultaneously on both the right and left sides of the brain, one half usually dominates over the other for a period of twenty-five to two-hundred minutes, then the other half takes over and dominates for awhile.

Recent research suggests that it is beneficial to be able to alter right and left brain dominance at will, thus augmenting their contribution to each other. For example, we may be better able to verbalize (left hemisphere function) our creativity (right hemisphere function).

However, the most beneficial state appears to be produced when the two sides of the brain are operating together in harmony. That is, thinking is produced by the whole brain acting as a single cohesive unit, instead of separately with the left or right side dominating at any time.

This whole brain thinking is associated with deep physical relaxation, serenity, mental clarity and promotion of high levels of mental functioning, which are states of consciousness associated with the alpha and theta brain waves.

Meditation has been found to induce this state of balance. In fact, researchers have observed that the more experienced and skillful the meditators, the more perfect the unity and the more quickly and consistently was this unity achieved.

Thus the purpose of meditation is to elevate consciousness by stimulating the whole brain to emit alpha (light meditative state) and ideally theta (deep meditative state) brain waves.

Once we know what these states feel like and how to achieve them, we become more able to think in alpha or theta states at any time at will.

The benefit of this ability to self-regulate thinking is not only feeling more relaxed and stress-free but also more creative, intuitive, and able to heal oneself and others. The physical benefits include better health and a longer, happier life.

Science is just beginning to understand and explain the exact nature of thoughts. What is known to date is that **our thoughts are concrete, permanent patterns** with which we create the blueprint for our entire life. **All** of our thoughts actively determine to the smallest detail what *happens* to us in life. The explanation for this phenomenon is beyond the scope of this book and is the subject of another. What is important here is to realize that whether we are consciously aware of it or not, our thoughts determine our life.

Our consciousness can be likened to a mirror in which our thoughts are reflected back to us as our destiny. For example, if we think we will fail, we attract failure, and if we think we will succeed, we actually bring about success.

> *Your world is a living expression of how you are*
> *using and have used your mind.*
> **Earl Nightingale**

Because there may be a delay, sometimes of years, between our thoughts and events in our life, we do not always associate our thoughts with the events. It is to our benefit to acquire this knowledge and to proceed accordingly.

If, after reading this book, you come away with nothing more than an understanding of the importance of your thoughts, you will have gained the key to all the beauty, happiness, and success you may desire.

CHAPTER

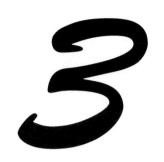

THOUGHTS AND FEELINGS

HOW THOUGHTS GENERATE
EMOTIONAL STATES AND FEELINGS

The association between our brain's electrical activity or thoughts and our emotional moods and feelings is the result of production and release of specific chemical substances by the brain nerve cells in response to being electrically stimulated by thoughts.

These brain chemicals or neurotransmitters are responsible for creating all our emotional states and feelings. Different thoughts produce very specific and exact mixtures of these brain chemicals which in turn produce very specific feelings. For example depression, anxiety, anger, distrust, faith, love and contentment are all the result of the effects caused by very specific mixtures of brain chemicals.

These in turn cause the production and release of other chemicals including hormones which in a cascading fashion influence not only the production of certain further thoughts and feelings but also affect the entire physical body directly, by means of the endocrine hormone and nervous systems.

THOUGHTS AND FEELINGS ARE INSEPARABLE

Since thoughts generate feelings, the two are inseparably linked.

The feelings then generate a whole range of other effects which potentially influence the whole body. Because of this great sphere of influence, it is the feeling that can charge the thought with power. Try the following experiment to demonstrate the power of feelings.

Say to yourself, "Lemons are sour." Now imagine biting into a lemon. Taste the sourness and smell the lemon as you bite into it. Your salivary glands will release saliva and your face will grimace as you feel the sour taste of the lemon. See how much more real the feeling makes the thought?

Now say, "I am beautiful" or "I am handsome." If you do not feel beautiful or handsome, this magnificent thought is nothing but a few words without power or effect. Feelings are discussed in more detail in Chapter 6.

Our thoughts can result in our feeling on top of the world when they are positive, or in the pit of depression when they are negative. That is, heaven and hell are states of mind.

THE EFFECTS OF THOUGHTS AND FEELINGS ON OUR BODY

The nature of our thoughts determines whether the feelings generated will be positive or negative and these in turn will have the equivalent effects on our body.

Only a small number of the chemical substances released in response to thoughts and feelings have been identified to date. The variety of our body's complex interactions both detrimental and healing, appears to be limitless.

Among these chemical substances are endorphins, which are similar to morphine. These substances, triggered for example by positive thoughts or exercise, give us a natural high. Unlike drugs taken externally, which are very harmful, the natural endorphins are beneficial to our body. They heal our feelings of dis-ease, by simulating positive feelings, and not only improve the quality of life but can also prolong life itself, a result of their beneficial physical effects.

This mechanism, for example, has been proposed as an explanation why in Biblical times people who lived in God, in this natural state of positivity guided by moral laws and commandments, were reputed to have lived extraordinarily long lives—as did Abraham and Sarah, despite a harsh environment where the average life expectancy was roughly thirty-five years.

The opposite is also true. Negative thoughts or lack of adherence to universally accepted lawful conduct lead not only to feeling bad (that is, emotional dis-ease) but also to actual physical disease. Research has shown that negative feelings such as depression, anger, and anxiety can suppress the immune system, by causing the release of certain harmful chemicals in our body, as well as the suppression of the beneficial substances.

Bad feelings have no nutritional value.

Henry Winkler

Suppression of the immune system makes us more vulnerable to infections, as well as to cancer. Anxiety and anger can also be associated with high blood pressure and can increase the risk of heart disease.

This release of chemicals in our body is why it is better to forgive, lest the resentment and anger hurt us by the release of harmful substances **in our own body**.

All we have to do is change our thinking to positive, constructive thoughts, and we will increase our sense of well being here and now because good feelings do have a positive nutritional value.

Proof of this beneficial effect of positive thoughts and actions has recently been provided by the Institute for the Advancement of Health, which found that people who performed volunteer work regularly for at least two hours, once a week, were ten times more likely to be in good health than those who didn't. Thus, healing ourselves and healing the world are inseparably interrelated.

We heal the world by healing our own mind.

Peter Azer

And we heal our own mind by helping to heal the world around us.

C H A P T E R

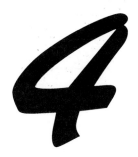

TAKING CONTROL OF OUR THOUGHTS

Sometimes if you want to see a change for the better, you have to take things into your own hands.

Clint Eastwood

WHY IT IS DIFFICULT TO CHANGE OUR HABITUAL PATTERNS OF THINKING

One of the difficulties in controlling thoughts is that they occur so rapidly that we may acquire the false impression that they are something which happens to us, something outside our control.

The other difficulty is that thoughts appear to produce permanent grooves or pathways in our brain which help subsequent thoughts of a similar nature travel along the pathways more easily. Thus, certain patterns of habitual thinking are established. It appears that in brain tissue, as well as other areas of our life:

The more deeply the path is etched, the more it is used, and the more it is used, the more deeply it is etched.

Jo Coudert

Confirming this hypothesis, Dr. Heath found that patients who suffered from painful emotional disorders such as suicidal depression, schizophrenia, violent rages and chronic intractable pain had an exaggerated ability to experience pain but little or no ability to experience pleasure.

These patients were able to alleviate their symptoms by having electrodes implanted in their brain, through which they stimulated their brains to experience pleasure instead of pain.

Dr. Heath concluded that:

> *Each system of the brain (pleasure and pain) is seemingly capable of overwhelming or inhibiting the other. Activation of the pleasure system by electrical stimulation eliminates signs and symptoms of emotional or physical pain, or both, and obliterates changes or recordings associated with the painful state.*

In other words, the pleasurable pathways can overcome or eliminate the grooves conducting electrical impulses or thoughts of pain.

Unfortunately, the opposite is also true. Habitually negative thinking can overwhelm occasional positive thoughts.

Our mind is constantly engaged in silent thinking or self-talk. If we are not in control of our self-talk we are at its mercy, feeling low when our thoughts happen to be negative. Fortunately, we can control what and how we think.

The most difficult and harmful negative thoughts are those sold to us as facts by those closest to us. Despite the fact that words such as "good," "bad," "fat," and "unattractive" are not facts and represent opinions and generalizations that often tell us more about the person speaking, the creation of permanent grooves would explain why such words can have a powerful effect on us, if we let them.

Dr. Chapman and his colleagues at the University of Rochester showed that distinct measurable brain electrical patterns were created in their subjects who thought of specific words such as "good," "bad," "beautiful," and "crime." This research suggests not only that the brain may have a universal brain wave language, but also that words themselves have the power to stimulate the brain to resonate along positive or negative pathways, depending on the words that we allow into our consciousness.

If we accept the negative terms and allow them to enter our consciousness, not only do we allow them to demean us, but, if our thinking is not guarded against their negative influence, even one negative word can initiate a whole avalanche of consequent negative thoughts.

For example, telling yourself "I am stupid" when you make a mistake, or "I am a failure" if you lose your job, can open up a vast number of negative pathways which can overwhelm you into thinking and feeling as though the whole of you is stupid or a failure, instead of focusing just on the action or event that led to those judgmental statements. The natural conclusion of thinking that you are totally stupid or a failure is that you are therefore, completely worthless; you'll be like that forever and there is no way out. Depressing thoughts indeed!

These kinds of thoughts lead to a feeling of hopelessness, helplessness, depression, and lack of control. They start a vicious cycle of decreasing self-esteem, more hopelessness, further lack of control, and so on.

Physiologically-based consequences of the way our brain functions lead to two important conclusions which can guard us against negative influences.

First is the need to select our environment, the people we interact with on a daily basis, very carefully.

> *We begin to see, therefore, the importance of selecting our environment with the greatest of care, because environment is the mental feeding ground out of which the food that goes into our minds is extracted.*
>
> **Napoleon Hill**

Secondly, and even more importantly, there is the need to control our own mind so it does not succumb to any external influence, which is not always under our direct control.

> *A singular strength of mind is required to enable a man to live among others consistently*

> *with his own ideas and convictions, to be master of himself and not fall into the habits or exhibit the same passions as those with whom he associates.*
>
> **Spinoza**

Unless of course these habits are themselves beneficial.

Despite initial appearances, the reality is that we can be in charge of our thoughts - if and when we choose. Destructive negative thinking patterns can be overcome and new beneficial, positive pathways created and reinforced by conscious choice.

This choice to think differently can be aided by associating the change, the new thoughts, with pleasure and reinforcing them by repetition.

However, before applying the power of our free will, we first need awareness of what needs to be changed.

AWARENESS

> *Every growth in awareness is, in the last analysis, a growth in self-awareness. What we observe in the world depends on our own **capacity** for observation. An anguished spirit will find in everything justification for its anguish. A joyous spirit will see reasons for gladness everywhere. No amount of pious maxims or lofty philosophy can bring light into man's world beyond what already exists in his own consciousness.*
>
> **J. Donald Walters**
> **(Kriyananda)**

The first step towards control is becoming aware of the internal dialogue, without repressing, denying, or negatively judging the self-talk. Just listen with an open heart. If we are unaware of our self-talk, we are unable to control it and are at its mercy, consequently feeling low when our thoughts are negative.

Only when we know what negative thinking has led to our present circumstances can we change our thinking for the better.

Understanding And Evaluation

Try to understand what originated your negative experience or feeling, being aware that although it may appear otherwise, painful feelings proceed from negative thoughts.

Are you feeling hurt because you have accepted someone's judgmental comments about you as a true reflection of who you are? When you understand where your negative thoughts originated, you can then make the conscious decision of either rejecting them or accepting them as true, in which case you have the choice of doing something about it.

Accepting Responsibility

The worst thing that could happen to us would be that someone else's comments or our own negative thoughts about ourselves might, in fact, be true. In that case, it would be better to accept the responsibility and do whatever we could to improve the situation.

Of course, taking responsibility and looking honestly at what we are doing to contribute to our own pain carries its own pain—the pain of truth about ourselves: that we may not be as wonderful as we would like to think we are. But truth is painful only in the short run. In the long run, it is considerably more painful and damaging to our self-esteem, to continue to pretend and defend the outer image of **false goodness or strength**, because deep down, sooner or later, we will sense our own fakery.

Letting go of our rosy picture of ourselves is not always easy. It means forsaking our personal point of view, which hurts our pride and vanity. Honesty takes courage but creates respect. If we are honest, we feel comfortable with ourselves. Feeling comfortable with ourselves builds true self-esteem, confidence, and security. This true strength of character is integrity.

Integrity is our most precious possession, for it is the only thing we truly possess. It is the essence of our belief in ourselves and therefore the true source of our inner personal power and effectiveness. Without belief in ourselves, we may be in possession of what is perceived as external sources of power, such as an attractive appearance, material possessions or social status. However all these become useless if, in situations of stress or difficulty, we crumble because of our lack of belief in ourselves.

Further, if we are not true to ourselves, we cannot be true to others. Adherence to truth is an inner law of our being, which determines all our actions and interactions with others. If we cannot trust ourselves, how can we trust anyone else and how can anyone else trust us?

Our adherence to truth is a reflection of how responsible we are. Truth is freedom; it releases us from bondage:

> *Bondage is...subjection to external influences*
> *and internal negative thoughts and attitudes.*
>
> **W. Clement Stone**

WILLINGNESS TO TAKE ACTION

Next comes the willingness to do something about changing any negative thinking. This may sound simple and easy. In fact it is a giant step when,

> *You will suddenly realize that the reason you*
> *never changed was because you didn't want to.*
>
> **Robert Schuller**

It is comforting to feel like a victim, to shift the responsibility for any unpleasant circumstances and painful feelings, to blame someone else for them instead of looking at what we are doing to create them in the first place.

> *To avoid blame we need to first ask ourselves*
> *what we contributed toward a difficulty or failure*
> *before looking for reasons outside ourselves.*

Life is not meant to be a struggle. We are not meant to suffer, and to continue to suffer is not a virtue. What is a virtue is to become aware of and to change the thinking that created the struggle and suffering in the first place, in accord with the universally operating law of cause and effect: whatever we put out into the world through our thoughts and actions will come back to us.

> *Sow much, reap much; sow little, reap little.*
>
> **Chinese Proverb**

> *Give and you'll be given. Be generous and life will be generous with you.*
>
> **Erwin Scheibner**

Are you happy with yourself and your life? Are there areas that would benefit from a change? If there are, then the next step is choice.

CONSCIOUS CHOICE

> *Our greatest power is the power to choose. We can decide where we are, what we do, and what we think. No one can take the power to choose away from us. It is ours alone. We can do what we want to do. We can be who we want to be.*
>
> **Wynn Davis**

Dr. Victor Frankl, through his own experiences in the Nazi concentration camps, demonstrated the ability of the human mind to transcend and thus survive even the most inconceivably inhuman cruelty.

Along with some of his fellow prisoners, Dr. Frankl made the decision to rise above his captive circumstances. And not only did he survive the ordeal, but also, discovered for himself and for the rest of us that,

> *Everything can be taken away from a man but one thing: the last of the human freedoms — to choose one's attitude in any given set of circumstances, to choose one's own way.*
>
> **Victor Frankl**

The stress Dr. Frankl was forced to endure and overcome, puts into perspective what we consider as stress. In comparison, our stresses are but minor irritations that sometimes, nevertheless, overwhelm us in our civilized Western society today.

If we ever feel overwhelmed to the point of saying, "I can't stand my life — I can't take it anymore", Dr. Frankl's book, *The Last of the Human Freedoms*, will broaden our perspective on our so-called "stresses" and will increase our faith and courage.

DETACHMENT

After we have become aware of, accepted the responsibility for our destructive thinking, and have decided to replace it with positive, constructive thoughts, detachment makes it easier to actually employ such constructive thinking on a daily basis. But to detach is not easy.

> *Detachment requires faith...in ourselves, in God,*
> *in other people, and in the natural order and des-*
> *tiny of things in this world.*
> **Melodie Beattie**

Detachment comes only after we see all our conscious thoughts and feelings: **without guilt, condemnation, or dwelling on our shortcomings, just recognition that they are there.**

At the same time, it is also crucial to remember that what we say and do is a reflection of us at that moment in time. Our thoughts and actions at any particular moment do not represent ALL that we are or are capable of being.

They are not the *entire* us, just a small part of us at that moment in time. **OUR POTENTIAL IS INFINITE.**

This is a very important distinction, for if we identify ourselves completely or even partly with what we do or **what we look like**, criticism of our action or appearance by anyone becomes a sentence of death, or at least, a painful, wounding experience to us personally.

WE NEED TO SEE OUR FAULTS BUT NOT IDENTIFY WITH THEM

Detachment means seeing ourselves as we are, and accepting the responsibility for it, but retaining the ability to change.

By not identifying with our thoughts and feelings, we retain the freedom of our infinite potential.

Seeing the truth about ourselves is best achieved by not taking it too personally, but detaching. Detachment saves us from the pain of negative emotions which invariably arise when our ideal image does not match the truth of reality.

For example, when someone asks whether we have put on weight, we have a choice of responses. We can say to ourselves,

Choice 1: They are right. I have put on ten pounds. I feel awful about it. I feel worthless and undesirable. No one will ever love me. I will always be lonely.

This response is not only accepting the truth of the observation but taking it further and allowing our own personal assessment of the undesirableness of being overweight to hurt and overwhelm us.

Choice 2: They are right. I have put on ten pounds. I don't like it, but I can do something about it.

This is a detached response. It does not deny the truth, but saves us the pain of any negative emotions.

Choice 3: I have put on ten pounds, but I am not willing to alter my lifestyle to lose this weight.

This is an acceptance of responsibility in a detached manner, without the baggage of negative emotions.

Detachment allows empathy to surface more easily. When we simply listen with empathy and compassion, we allow our and others' true thoughts and feelings to surface.

Remaining silent and calm allows us to open our heart instead of engaging in a defensive reaction that leads to a power struggle.

Allow yourself to be vulnerable, to experience the emotion. Vulnerability is powerful, not weak, as it carries the power of honesty. Truth and reason will always triumph over their opposites.

> *When you are in pain or hurt, what you really want from others is for them to listen to you, be gentle with you and understand that you are upset. You do not want them to withdraw and get defensive. You do not want them to get upset with you when you are angry, but instead to recognize*

that you have been hurt...What you really want them to do is say, "Yes, I see. I am sorry I hurt you."...What they want from you is for you to love them.

Sanaya Roman

That includes ourselves. When we are in pain, our heart may be crying out for more love. Psychological pain indicates there is a difference between what we want and what we perceive we are getting. What we perceive we are not getting is usually lacking in ourselves, and (vice versa) what we perceive we are getting (both positive and negative) is usually present in ourselves. All we have to do is meet the want ourselves.

CHAPTER

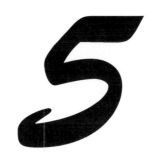

CHANGING THINKING PATTERNS

IDENTIFYING DISTORTED THINKING PATTERNS

To help eliminate destructive thinking, it is valuable to become familiar with several varieties of distorted thinking.

In his book, *Feeling Good*, Dr. David Burns defines ten types of negative, distorted thinking patterns. The following definitions are quoted from his book.

1. *All-or-nothing thinking — you see things in black and white categories. If your performance falls short of perfect, you see yourself as a total failure.*

Example: You are on a diet and have just eaten some cookies. You say to yourself: "I have eaten half a box of cookies already. I might as well eat the rest since I can't diet anyway. I'll always be fat."

2. *Overgeneralization: You see a single negative event as a never-ending pattern of defeat.*

Example: "I have eaten half a box of cookies. I have totally failed my diet. I have no will power."

3. *Mental filter: You pick out a single detail and dwell on it exclusively so that your vision of all reality becomes darkened, like a drop of* black ink *that discolors the entire beaker of water.*

Example: You have a job you like. You do not complete a task your employer requested you to do. He expresses his disapproval. You say to yourself: "I am being reprimanded for one little thing?! Who does my boss think he is? He never appreciates what I do for him. I resent him for being judgmental and critical."

4. *Disqualifying the positive: You reject positive experiences by insisting they 'don't count' for some reason or other. In this way you can maintain a negative belief that is contradicted by your everyday experiences.*

Example: Your boss gives you a compliment. You think: "She always criticizes everything I do. Why is she so nice to me now? She probably just wants something."

5. *Jumping to conclusions: You make a negative interpretation even though there are no definite facts that convincingly support your conclusions.*

a. Mind-reading. You arbitrarily conclude that someone is reacting negatively to you and you don't bother to check this out.

b. The Fortune Teller error. You anticipate that things will turn out badly and you feel convinced that your prediction is an already-established fact.

Example: You go to a party and the person you are talking to does not appear to be listening to you. You think: "He doesn't like me. He is purposefully ignoring me. How rude. Well, I don't like him either. I don't fit here. No one here will like me, I hate parties, they're so boring. It's a waste of time being here." He thinks, "I hope she likes me. I wish I wasn't so shy."

6. *Magnification (catastrophizing) or minimization. You exaggerate the importance of things (such as your goofup or someone else's achievement), or you inappropriately shrink things until they appear tiny (your own desirable qualities or other fellow's imperfections). This is also called the binocular trick.*

Example: You give a presentation of an action plan at work. Your boss responds by accepting a portion of your ideas, modifying some and rejecting others. Your co-worker, Sandy, gives one also and more of her ideas are accepted. You respond: "I gave a terrible presentation. Nothing was acceptable. I will probably lose my job. I am not as creative as Sandy. She is much smarter than me. I feel like a failure."

7. *Emotional Reasoning: You assume that your negative emotions necessarily reflect the way things really are: 'I feel it, therefore, it must be true.'*

Example: Your boss does not agree with all your ideas. You, therefore, think that nothing you do is good enough. He says: "I like most of your ideas. Some are not appropriate, I think, for the market we are trying to reach." You think: "He is judgmental and critical. I feel he hates me. I put in 110% and this is all I get!"

8. *Should statements: You try to motivate yourself with 'shoulds' and 'shouldn'ts,' as if you had to be whipped and punished before you could be expected to do anything. 'Musts' and 'oughts' are also offenders. The emotional consequence is guilt. When you direct should statements toward others, you feel anger, frustration and resentment.*

Example: "I should visit my in-laws at Christmas time, even though I don't like them and don't enjoy myself," **and** "If I work hard, my boss should be appreciative. He should also appreciate and encourage my ideas. If I am nice to him, he should be nice to me."

This certainly sounds fair and reasonable but does not work like that in the reality of our present life. People will act and react according to their (spiritual) maturity, regardless of how well we treat them or pay them.

'Should' statements are particularly difficult to eliminate. They are based on the false assumption that even after childhood, people are obligated to continue to meet our needs, and if they don't, there is something wrong with them and we have the right to get mad and express our anger because this is what we as humans are entitled to do.

9. *Labeling and mislabeling: This is an extreme form of overgeneralization. Instead of describing your error, you attach a negative label to yourself: 'I'm a loser.' When someone else's behavior rubs you the wrong way, you attach a negative label to him: 'He's nothing but a critical and judgmental tyrant.' Mislabeling involves describing an event with language that is highly colored and emotionally loaded.*

Example: Your husband is outspoken about the children's misbehavior. You disagree with him and say: "You are nothing but a tyrant! You are mean and authoritarian. You always have to be right."

10. *Personalization: You see yourself as the cause of some negative external event for which, in fact, you were not primarily responsible.*

Example: You had a friend over for dinner. You did not serve any alcohol. On the way home, he has an accident. You think: "It's all my fault. If I hadn't invited him for dinner he wouldn't have had the accident."

In addition to these categories, there are three others which warrant a mention:

1. Superstitious thinking: our culture abounds in superstitions. We outgrow stepping on cracks, but there is still Friday the thirteenth. Some people believe that bad things happen to good people and that these unfortunate events are proof of their goodness; or, that it is better to expect a negative outcome to avoid being disappointed.

2. Hypocritical thinking: thinking that lacks integrity. For example, believing that attending church and saying one loves God will automatically excuse all behavior. That suppression of negative feelings by positive affirmations is enough to overcome difficulties and rationalizing any problems as being simply the will of God, instead of looking at the reasons for the failure or difficulty and doing something actively constructive about it.

3. Limited thinking: thinking bridled with limitation can be so insidious that a whole lifetime can go by before realizing how a potentially infinitely successful life has been one wasted by self-imposed failure, unhappiness and missed opportunities. Limited thinking is based on the false premise that external circumstances and obstacles are greater than our ability to overcome them. It reflects a thinking of powerlessness, of lack of faith in one's personal effectiveness and lack of courage to overcome external obstacles. When phrases such as: "I can't," "it won't work," "it can't be done," "it will only work if it's done in this specific way" come to mind, we need to remember:

> *...if you have faith as small as a mustard seed...Nothing will be impossible for you.*
> **Matthew 17:20**

The subject of not accepting limitation is one that is particularly close to my heart. I was born in Czechoslovakia, a country where self-imposed limitation is an accepted way of life. It was abhorred by my parents whose life, even under the communist regime, exemplified a refusal to submit to limitation imposed by any destructive negative outward circumstances.

It is their example that lead me to break away from the traditional methods of treatment and develop not only laser techniques that eliminated scarring for the treatment of portwine birthmarks and other blood vessel malformations in the early 1980s, but also, not to accept that scars were permanent and to develop further more recent laser techniques to stimulate our body to improve or remove scars.

The irrational nature of limitation was highlighted during my recent visit to Czechoslovakia, which now consists of two separate countries.

In the capital of Slovakia, the elevators in the main department store take people only up, they "can't" take them down. The customers have to walk down twelve flights of stairs, while the operators go down with the empty elevators.

When asked why one can not go down in the elevators, the answer was "because it's impossible, it's always been like that and there is nothing we can do about it. We can't take you down. You have to walk."

No wonder communism, which is itself a philosophy based on limiting the human potential and stifling creativity, took such a long time to break down and is back in those countries where people don't know how to cope with self-reliance and responsibility.

It takes courage to depart from the traditional and generally accepted way of thinking or doing something – of risking rejection and standing alone in the face of breaking with tradition and taking the uncertain road of not accepting limitation. To overcome limitation takes spiritual fortitude.

> *Heroism works in contradiction to the voice of*
> *mankind, and in contradiction, for a time, to the*
> *voice of the "great" and "good." Heroism is an obe-*

> *dience to a secret impulse of an individuals charac-*
> *ter.*
>
> **Emerson**

And heroism is:

> *...the brilliant triumph of the soul over the flesh,*
> *that is to say, over fear of any kind, fear of poverty,*
> *of suffering, of doubt about one's abilities...There is*
> *no serious piety without heroism. Heroism is the*
> *dazzling and glorious concentration of courage.*
>
> **Amiel**

Nothing Is Impossible

There is a solution to every problem. Just because *we* do not see a solution at this moment in time, does not mean one does not exist.

Who invented airplanes? Not the men who thought they could not fly.

The raw materials to build airplanes and all the modern comforts which we take for granted today were present in the Stone Age. So, where did all the modern miracles come from? They originated with an idea in the mind of someone who was not subject to self-imposed limitation. It was only after the ideas were conceived that they were materialized into reality.

> *The secret of making something work in our*
> *lives is, first of all, the deep desire to make it work.*
>
> *Then, the faith and belief that it can work.*
>
> *Then, to hold that clear definite vision in your*
> *consciousness and see it working out step-by-step,*
> *without one thought of doubt or disbelief.*
>
> **Eileen Caddy**

It is very worthwhile to become familiar with the various types of thought distortions, so as to recognize them and avoid them in our thinking patterns. I would also encourage you to read Dr. Burns book *Feeling Good* to help with any misconceptions in thinking and feeling, as well as some of the others listed in the bibliography.

ELIMINATING DISTORTED THINKING PATTERNS

Once we have identified any negative thinking patterns, and detached them from the totality of who we are, the next step is eliminating them.

The best way to eliminate all thoughts of limitation, lack, or poverty of any kind is by replacing these harmful thoughts with constructive, positive thinking. The same way we can dislodge ice floating on top of water in a cup: by pouring in more water.

However, overcoming the habit of negative thinking patterns is not easy. It takes a great deal of determined self-discipline to permanently change old habits of negative thinking and feeling.

Self-discipline is effective self-management. It comes from within and requires subordination of thoughts, feelings, and desires, in favor of the chosen goal or ideal.

The ideal of peace of mind and quality life for all is well worth the effort of dedicated application of will power day to day and moment to moment to accomplish this objective.

The subordination of our impulsive thinking, which at the time may appear to be easier, in favor of any longer term ideal, is the price we pay for success. It is also our reward for the sacrifice. In fact, self-discipline means we love and respect ourselves.

> *No discipline seems pleasant at the time, but painful. Later on, however, it produces a harvest of righteousness* and peace to those who have been trained by it.*
>
> **Hebrews 12:11**

The key to overcoming the habit of inertia is to actively **make** ourselves replace negative or destructive thoughts with positive thoughts, even if we don't feel like it. Such effort is a valuable asset that is amply rewarded.

> *The successful person has the habit of doing things failures don't like to do.*
>
> **E.M. Gray**

---

* In the Bible *righteousness* refers to principled, ethical or right thinking.

> *The kind of people I look for to fill manage-*
> *ment spots are the eager beavers, the mavericks.*
> *These are the guys who try to do more than they're*
> *expected to do — they always reach.*
>
> **Lee Iacocca**

To create this kind of will power, decide to do something you thought you couldn't do. Choose a simple task at first. Don't overwhelm yourself by choosing tasks that take longer than about fifteen minutes.

For example, make yourself exercise for fifteen minutes a day. After the first few times of making yourself do it, you will derive pleasure from the activity, enough to continue your daily exercise without having to talk yourself into it. Refuse to give up, and master one thing at a time. Don't dissipate your energies by jumping to another activity before completing the one you set out to do.

Or better still, decide to undertake something that requires even less time, like washing off your make-up and applying a moisturizer *every* night, no matter how tired you are. You will be amazed how breaking through the inertia barrier even in such a mundane way will help you start and complete more complex and time-consuming activities.

Regarding constructive thinking, determine to become aware of any distorted thinking habits and to change them one day at a time.

If we were to wait for the moment of inspiration and motivation to arrive, we would be waiting forever. It is action itself that inspires and motivates us to do more.

Action motivates, inaction stagnates.

Also, engaging yourself in action distracts you from any possible negative self-talk and empowers you with a sense of mastery that disproves the distorted thinking patterns.

> *Perhaps the most valuable result of all educa-*
> *tion is the ability to make yourself do the thing you*
> *have to do when it ought to be done, **whether you***
> ***like it or not,*** it is the first lesson that ought to be*
> *learned, and however early a man's training*

---

* bold type added

begins, it is probably the last lesson he learns thor-
oughly.

Thomas Huxley

What you will find is that when you actually do the task or change your negative thinking, it is not as unpleasant as you thought it was going to be, and you actually enjoy the task and reap the benefit of the newly acquired sense of self-esteem and well-being.

In my own experience, I was fortunate enough to have parents who not only taught me through their own example but also made me exercise will power at a very young age, both in thoughts and actions .

My parents are both geologists, and from the time I was about three years old, they would take me on their geological excursions to the mountains. They encouraged me to walk on my own, despite protestations that my legs were sore and I was thirsty.

At the time, I thought they were mean when they refused to carry me whenever I requested it. In retrospect, it's clear my parents showed me I could make it through my barriers of sore legs and anger at not having my desire of being carried met. They helped me transform my frustration at a very early age to thoughts, feelings and experience of self-mastery and exhilaration: I could and did make it.

I actually began to enjoy the walking and felt very proud of my achievements in self-discipline. Walking up mountains was especially difficult, for if you kept on looking up, the peak seemed to be rising higher and higher, and the distance already covered seemed minuscule compared to the distance yet to be covered.

My parents taught me the secret of climbing mountains and attaining any goal: you look down at the ground and put all your attention to every step and breath you take, not looking up except to see in what direction you are going. You harmonize your breathing with the walking. This way, you actually begin to enjoy the movement and rhythm of every step and breath; before you realize it, you have completed your task and you are at the top.

I have applied this very same principle to everything I have ever undertaken. At times, pushing myself through inertia-sparking thoughts like, "I don't feel like doing this now, I'll do it later," to enjoying the task at hand.

I remember my mother's advice: "If it's not fun, **make** it fun. Period." If it's not fun, don't do it, did not exist for my mother. She **made everything** she did fun by becoming totally absorbed and interested in the task.

Her direction of purposeful and complete concentration on the task at hand, from washing dishes to reading a book, created the situation and feeling of doing the work or activity purely for its own sake; for the joy of the movement, the performance of the task, while completely forgetting about any possible material or emotional benefits of the final result while the task was in progress.

Watching my parents work was like watching a ballet performance put on by the dancers for the pure joy of the dance. They made any work look fun, easy, and effortless.

Lasting material and especially spiritual rewards are a side benefit of positive thinking, guided by universal principles of correct ethical conduct and inspired by creative intuition.

Paradoxically, although it is not the purpose of such thinking to acquire material rewards, such thinking is precisely what **is** required to gain material wealth. Those who have acquired disciplined, intuitive wisdom are sought after in all fields of endeavor.

The greatest gift that your parents can give to you and the greatest gift that you can, in turn, give to your children and yourself, is encouragement to apply self-disciplined will power in all constructive thoughts and activities.

PERSEVERANCE THROUGH REPETITION

Perseverance is loyalty to our principles, our dreams, our ideals, and duty to ourselves and others whatever the task at hand. Perseverance is what allows us to overcome any obstacle. The only insurmountable obstacle that could arise comes from within: loss of the will to keep trying.

Any negative habit can be overcome by will power applied for as long as necessary to eliminate the negative habit and replace it with a positive one.

"Loyalty," my great spiritual teacher used to say, "is the first law of God. Most people are fickle.

They change their jobs, their spouses, their friends, their beliefs, their ideas — not because of any new expansion of awareness, but because they lack the simple power of perseverance.

One must be loyal to one's principles, and not allow oneself to be ruled by sentiment. To be loyal to others, and to one's assumed goals in life — not for sentimental reasons, but in the name of principle — is the way of divine progress. Perseverance can be difficult, for in every undertaking there is a certain amount of dull routine. Don't be ruled, therefore, by likes and dislikes, but do whatever has to be done. If it is right, let nothing intervene until the job is finished."

> **Paramahansa Yogananda**
> **as quoted by J. Donald Walters**
> **(Kriyananda)**

We achieve to the degree that we overcome the negative. Achievers are willing to pay the price of achievement. They sacrifice, struggle, work on, perhaps alone, weary and discouraged, and yet at each step overcome the negative. Overcoming the negative is the price of achievement — the price of greatness.

> **Wynn Davis**

Try, try, try, and keep on trying. Don't ever let anything interfere with your determination to accomplish what you set out to do, especially when you set out to change destructive negative thinking patterns and replace them with constructive positive thoughts.

C H A P T E R

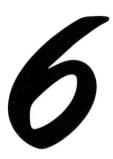

FEELING BEAUTIFUL

HOW WE FEEL IS MORE IMPORTANT THAN HOW WE LOOK, AND HOW WE FEEL DEPENDS ON HOW WE THINK

Feelings determine how we perceive the quality of our life. If we are feeling bad, our life will be perceived as such.

Feelings are like the color filter in glasses — through feelings, we can either view the world as a wonderful place to be in or an unbearable place of deprivation and suffering.

The choice is ours.

Although it may appear otherwise, how we feel does depend on how we think. Negative thoughts *precede* the feeling of depression or any other painful emotion.

It is therefore important to be able to identify our painful or negative feelings and use them to find the faulty thinking patterns.

FEELINGS ARE NOT FACTS

Remember, it is what we really believe that matters. A report about something may be quite

> *untrue, but if you believe it, it has the same effect*
> *upon you as if it were true; and that again will*
> *depend upon the quality of feeling attached to it.*
>
> Emmet Fox

Distorted thoughts produce a very powerful illusion or appearance of truth reinforced by powerful emotions which also appear a true reflection of reality. This is so because the abnormal emotions *feel* as valid and real as the genuine feelings resulting from undistorted thoughts.

Unless we become aware of the distortion in our thinking and are able to identify and separate the abnormal versus the genuine feelings, we become caught in a vicious cycle of our own making. The abnormal feelings themselves lead to further distorted thoughts and consequent inappropriate actions which not only reinforce each other but gather momentum, creating a self-perpetuating vicious cycle.

Once caught in this vicious cycle, we come under its black spell which is very difficult to break even when we ourselves are aware of it, let alone when we are unaware of the distorted thinking that originated it.

It is even more difficult to reach and reason with someone else caught in this black magic trance created by distorted thoughts. Any input, especially pointing out the distorted thinking, only encourages further distorted thoughts by putting the person on the defensive, so that they further reinforce and justify their position. The result is not constructive as it only magnifies the consequent abnormal thoughts and feelings.

This is why it is virtually impossible to try to *change* another person, no matter how genuinely we may care about them or want them to change their unhappy, negative or destructive outlook on life. We can do nothing if their thinking is distorted even in some of the ways outlined in Chapter 5, and they are unaware and unwilling to see and change their distorted thinking themselves.

Depression is a particularly powerful and destructive emotion which can result from any one or a number of the distorted thinking patterns. Because of its powerful influence on all aspects of life, it can wreak major devastation in our work and personal life.

> *The mental prison is an illusion, a hoax you*
> *have inadvertently created, but it **seems** real*
> *because it **feels** real.* *

David Burns

In India, they catch small monkeys by putting a banana in a cage with bars wide enough to allow a monkey to get through but not the banana held sideways to the bars. Once a monkey grabs hold of the banana, he refuses to let go and is caught — even though he could easily escape and be free if only he would let go of the banana.

What bananas are you holding onto?

Believing in the reality of our distorted thoughts and feelings is just like getting hold of a banana and thus becoming a prisoner, when all we have to do is simply let go of our self-imposed and self-perpetuating prison of distorted thinking.

What is the key to let yourself out of your emotional prison?

> *Simply this: Your thoughts create your emo-*
> *tions; therefore, your emotions cannot prove that*
> *your thoughts are accurate. Unpleasant feelings*
> *merely indicate that you are thinking something*
> *negative and believing it. Your emotions follow*
> *your thoughts just as surely as baby ducks **follow***
> *their mother. But the fact that the baby ducks fol-*
> *low faithfully along doesn't prove that the mother*
> *knows where she is going!*

David Burns

The reason for this powerful illusion is the way our conscious mind works. Look at the following diagram. You will likely see it in one of two ways.

* bold type added

You will see the diagram either as a white swirl on a black background or as a black swirl on a white background. It is difficult to see both as background at the same time.

This tendency to concentrate on just one aspect at any one time is the very nature of our conscious mind. If our mind were constantly distracted by each new input from other aspects of the conscious or unconscious mind, we would be unable to concentrate and unable to carry out a single task.

Thus, as soon as we allow our conscious mind to entertain or focus on negative thoughts, it can no longer focus on positive thoughts. Like the monkey, when it is focused on the banana, he is unable to see the freedom of letting go of the banana.

IDENTIFYING THE MOST COMMON UNPLEASANT FEELINGS

Just as it is worthwhile to familiarize ourselves with the various types of distorted thinking, so it is worthwhile to familiarize ourselves with the various types of distorted feelings. Identifying and understanding these can help us to eliminate them. The most common destructive feelings are anger, depression, fear and doubt.

ANGER

The ability to express anger strongly has a very important survival value. According to Dr. William Glasser, anger is one of the most powerful behavioral mechanisms we have to affect our environment. It is particularly useful and powerful for manipulating our environment during the dependent years of our childhood.

In some situations, even after we grow up and can take care of ourselves, anger is appropriate and useful. Just as red lights safeguard our safety on the road, so anger makes us aware that we are in a situation that may not be in our best interest. It has become popular to teach that because anger is an unpleasant and destructive emotion it is better not to have it at all. This sentiment is often used as a form of manipulation by people who want all their behavior, which they impose on others, excused as being okay, regardless of the effect their behavior has on others.

When the people who are being used react with understandable and appropriate anger, the users will attempt to control them with guilt and a false self-righteous attitude; pointing out that anger is bad and therefore if a person reacts even to unreasonable behavior with anger, they too are bad and the real user is thus not only superior but entitled to get away with whatever they impose on the other person.

When human nature develops or matures enough that we no longer need traffic lights because traffic will run smoothly simply by perfect cooperation, we will no longer have the need for anger as a warning and teaching tool either. We can contribute toward such enlightened behavior by learning as quickly as possible what anger has to teach us.

That is, anger is a warning signal that serves to protect us against intentional or unintentional harm by others as well as ourselves. It is only when anger does not achieve the desired goal of self-protection that it becomes counterproductive. For example, when in self-defense we become angry with another who in turn becomes angry and retaliates in a fashion that further hurts us or takes advantage of us, our anger is not productive.

Because the feeling of anger floods and overwhelms our body very quickly, most of the time we do not realize that we are making a **choice** to be angry.

> *When you are feeling depreciated, angry or drained, it is a sign that other people are not open to your energy.*
> **Sanaya Roman**

The reciprocal of this situation is that,

> *...if you fail to act in a manner that takes into account the feelings and interests of others, you are likely to end up less happy because sooner or later they will retaliate when they notice you are taking advantage of them.*
> **David Burns**

This retaliation takes the form of anger. We may even be angry with ourselves for taking advantage of or not appreciating some part of ourselves.

As infants and children, we are totally dependent on our caretakers. However, it is a normal and a necessary process of growing up that we become less dependent on others and more able to take care of and meet our own needs. People who are not completely mature continue to have the expectation that their needs should continue to be met without their contribution matching the requirements of the situation.

The expectation of having ones needs met and not being expected to meet other's needs, or feeling of entitlement, which was the situation in childhood, perpetuated into adulthood, leads to most of our problems in relating to ourselves and others.

It results in a feeling of being treated unfairly, which causes anger to be experienced as a "**moral emotion**," writes Dr. David Burns in his book *Feeling Good*, "you will be extremely hesitant to let go of that righteous feeling. You will have the nearly irresistible urge to defend and justify your anger with **religious zeal**. Overcoming this will require an act of great will power, and a willingness to think as an adult and put oneself in the shoes of the other, to empathize and to be willing to adjust accordingly."

As we grow up and come to realize that not all our needs will be met, we learn to not only meet some of our own needs but those of others around us. Exchanging our meeting others needs for them meeting ours becomes a more positive way of fulfilling what we want than simply demanding them without reciprocating.

However, the *expectation* of reciprocating creates further problems, because it creates an unspoken **hidden demand** which is even more powerful and therefore better able to manipulate others and ourselves to meet our demands.

Applied to all human relationships it says:

> If I do nice things for people, they **should** recip-
> rocate and I am entitled to this response.

This certainly sounds fair and reasonable and the world would be a better place if everyone always thought and acted in integrity, treating others in the same way they want to be treated themselves.

Unfortunately, this is not always so in practice, not only because integrity requires strength of character and its moment to moment application of ethical and moral principles in all aspects of life, but also because people are different. These differences in needs and desires mean that relationships are rarely automatically or perfectly reciprocal at all times.

Good relationships require continued effort from all parties concerned by means of effective communication, empathy, being willing to see the other's point of view, to give and to compromise. They require a willingness to admit to being wrong and to adjust accordingly. In other words, a willingness to be vulnerable, to change and to grow.

Empathy is probably the greatest asset and the most important ingredient in good relationships. It is the ability to think with an open heart and embrace the other person by stepping outside our own feelings and into theirs. It requires our willingness to *experience* what the other person feels and experiences and thus be able to reach a mutually agreeable solution through understanding while maintaining reverence for *all* parties involved.

> *Do not make the other person, or yourself wrong. If you want a healing connection with others, know how much to give, and how much to receive.*
>
> **Sanaya Roman**

Anger can be a very powerful teaching tool. If we listen to the thoughts and feelings that led to anger, we can learn the lesson we are being presented. For example, if we are angry about giving more than we are receiving, we can question why we are placing ourselves in such an unbalanced situation. Is it because we do not appreciate our giving, and therefore ourselves, enough?

> *These connections are messages from the universe telling you to pay attention to what you are doing to yourself, to look at ways you may be giving away your energy to those who cannot receive it. I call them reminders.*
>
> **Sanaya Roman**

Alternatively, we may be using anger in self-defense to cover up not giving enough to others.

WHY WE CONVERT ANGER INTO DEPRESSING AND CHOOSE MISERY OVER HAPPINESS

Anger is a straight forward emotion that occurs and overwhelms us rapidly and fades away just as quickly. Thus, as all babies discover sooner or later, anger is not always effective in getting our needs met. In fact, when used frequently over time, anger loses its effectiveness since the caretakers and those around us become used to the outbursts and either ignore them or laugh at them.

At about age two, children learn to use another emotion which is even more powerful in controlling others and getting what they want. According to David Glasser, this emotional tool is the act of "depressing." Instead of throwing a temper tantrum, they become sad, listless, and unresponsive. Most caretakers respond to this heart-wrenching behavior by giving the child attention and trying to cheer him up by giving him what he wants.

There is but one major problem with playing this role of a sad victim. **It is very painful**.

"Even when it works," writes Dr. Glasser in his book, *Control Theory*, "it is much more painful than angering. But it is so powerful and controlling of those around him (referring to a two-year-old child), he decides the pain is worth it and begins to use it frequently when he is frustrated. He also discovers that he must actually use the behavior **and** feel the pain. If he only pretends to depress and does not pay the price of the pain, people see through him, and it does not work."

Dr. Glasser goes on to describe how acting sad and depressed serves several functions. As he notes in *Control Theory*, the purposes of depressing are:

1. "To keep angering under control." Expressing excessive or too frequent anger can become counterproductive or even physically dangerous as our crime figures indicate.

2. "To get others to help us." Depressing makes it easier for us to ask for assistance by appealing to others' sympathy for us in our

unhappy or difficult situation. It is one of the most powerful means of asking for help without losing face as the request is not direct but hidden from both parties by an implicit denial that help is really needed. Camouflaging the request in this fashion makes it possible to maintain pseudo self-esteem by being able to maintain a veneer of not really needing the help.

3. "To excuse our unwillingness to do something more effective." It is tempting and appears to be easier to use pain and misery as an excuse for being ineffective or not facing a fearful situation.

4. "To gain powerful control" over the people we are attempting to influence. Appealing to the positive, sympathetic aspects of human nature is a very powerful means of getting others to do what we want, even if this may not be in their best interest. People are basically good. Most are genuinely willing to be helpful or at least want to appear to be so. To refuse a request for help, places a person in a very difficult position of appearing callous or not "good." It is understandable that an individual can thus be manipulated to succumb to the control of another, if they allow themselves to perceive their goodness and value to be at stake if they refuse to help. This is especially so for people who were manipulated in this fashion by their families during their childhood.

A healthy self-esteem is required to see through and to overcome such attempts at control.

Despite the fact that depressing, angering, anxieting, worrying, obsessing, guilting or any other such negative emotion is very powerful in controlling others, especially those who themselves are open to be manipulated by such tactics, the use of all these behaviors is an admission and a display of personal powerlessness. It reflects feelings of ineffectiveness in being able to deal with the circumstances and to communicate openly, directly, and effectively.

The use of such excess, but masked forcefulness, may temporarily result in gaining control indirectly, but it also carries the heavy price of perpetuating and voluntarily reinforcing the position of disempowerment which has the long-term consequences of damaging our sense of worth or self-esteem.

Day to day living involves confronting many frustrations. To overcome any obstacle we need to develop and use courage derived from the strength of our thinking guided by reason, moral principles, compassion and integrity which over time build and determine our character.

One of the reasons why it is difficult to give up these negative behaviors is precisely because they are so powerful. Which of these we choose, whether headaching, fretting or being a martyr depends on what we learned to work best for us in our life situations.

None are beneficial to us in the long run as all undermine our true strength. Self-worth comes from relying on ourselves. It is the psychological and spiritual *muscle*, which like our physical muscle, develops as a result of stimulation or exercise. Psychological and spiritual strengths develop as a consequence of the exercise of overcoming adversity through our own direct effort.

True empowerment does not come from controlling others. It comes from the effort of cultivating awareness and through discernment being able to control our thoughts, feelings and actions so we can always be confident in being able to rely on ourselves. It is the result of the courage to stand alone in the face of all odds.

Throughout the ages, true empowerment was and remains a side benefit of overcoming life's challenges, whatever they may be, in a spirit of courage and heroism.

> *Self-strength comes from relying on oneself. Not on reputation nor on wealth nor on the power of the law nor on any outward appearances, but on our own strength ... for this is the only thing which makes us men free.*
>
> Epictetus

Fear And Doubt

Finding your direction.

The purpose of growth is to become better. Accept your life as a gift. Accept the responsibility to act in your own best interests. Believe that if you

*are a good person, what you seek for yourself will
also be good for others, providing you are honest
about your needs.*

*Whenever people avoid acting in their own best
interests and shirk the responsibility for their lives,
they hold others ransom, demanding appreciation,
fulfillment and a sense of completeness by proxy.
The truth is that no one can ever fulfill you, except
you. The way you do that is to take risks. Failure
to do this is an act of fear and in the long run harmful to everyone.*

David Viscott

Take the risk of being responsible for your life.

According to the dictionary definition, fear is "a painful feeling of
impending danger, evil, trouble," and so on.

The feeling of fear is preceded by doubt. Fear is one of the most
serious and destructive negative feelings, since it can undermine and
destroy the potential of a whole lifetime.

Fear, like anger, has a survival purpose. It makes us aware of an
impending danger to our well-being. However, life, lived to the full,
does involve taking risks.

Our perception of the degree of risk and our ability to cope with it
determines how fearful we feel. Admitting fear is not cowardly. On the
contrary, it indicates strength:

*What is needed, rather than running away or
controlling or suppressing, or any other resistance,
is understanding fear; that means, watch it, learn
about it, come directly into contact with it. We are
to learn about fear, not how to escape from it....*

J. Krishnamurti

We are afraid only when we are not in harmony with ourselves.
When we do not face reality with honesty and courage and see ourselves as we really are; not as we would like to be perceived, but are
not that way in reality, because our thoughts and actions do not back
up the "nice" picture we have of ourselves.

That is, we either possess healthy self-esteem or low or pseudo self-esteem. **Constructive, positive thoughts and feelings bear the fruit of healthy self-esteem.**

> *A healthy self-esteem is valuing ourselves — seeing our strengths and weaknesses without feeling threatened.*

Healthy self-esteem enables us to look reality squarely in the face, to see our mistakes as we make them. Not merely justifying or defending ourselves, but using our intelligence fully to identify the facts of any situation and find **solutions** to any problems, even — and especially — if we are responsible for causing them.

Self-Esteem Is The Foundation Of All Human Success

Self-esteem and faith are two essential ingredients in the transformation of thoughts into their corresponding results in the material world.

Healthy or true self-esteem takes both positive and negative thoughts and together with faith transforms these into success.

Pseudo or low self-esteem either entertains negative thoughts or does not discern adequately between positive and negative or destructive thoughts. It transforms these into failure or only partial success.

Perhaps the most in-depth and succinct analysis of the causes, consequences, and solutions to the feelings of fear I have found is in two books: Dr. David Viscott's book, *Risking*, and Dr. Nathaniel Brandon's book, *The Psychology of Self-Esteem*. Both volumes are well worth reading. As Dr. Brandon points out, self-esteem is a sense of personal efficacy and personal worth. It consists of self-confidence and self-respect. "It is the conviction that one is competent to live and worthy of living."

We are not born with self-esteem — we acquire it by using our mind to reason and to deal with reality, and by using our power to choose, based on universal principles of right thinking (true righteousness) discussed in Chapter 8.

By using our mind to deal with the realities of life, we acquire a sense of control over our day-to-day existence. This gives us a sense of self-confidence and mastery and is the normal process of growing up from a helpless infant to a competent, mature adult.

It does not mean that we can never make a mistake or that we avoid situations for fear of making a mistake. On the contrary, true self-esteem is based on the conviction that despite fear and despite making mistakes in the past, we can rely on our ability to reason, evaluate, intuit and apply our knowledge and experience to act with competence and to correct our mistakes no matter how many times we have tried and not succeeded in the past.

In other words, it is the faith that we are competent in principle, not just in carrying out a particular task that we may be particularly good at; it is the faith in our general ability to deal with whatever reality we are confronted with.

The process of acquiring self-esteem begins in childhood. It is a process, not an achievement, that requires continual sustenance throughout our lives.

One of the first things we need to learn in childhood, so we can begin to build and then continue to sustain our self-esteem throughout our adult life, is that feelings and desires alone are not appropriate or adequate guides to what we do or how we behave. That is, just because we feel like doing something, is not in itself a proof or adequate reason for doing it.

The opposite is also true, if we are afraid or doubt our ability to perform a task, it does not mean that we ought to let these feelings alone stop us from doing it. In other words:

> *Emotions are not tools of knowing nor criteria of judgement.*
>
> Nathaniel Brandon

Self-esteem requires that we direct our actions by basing them on reasoned thinking and ethical principles, not on our feelings of the moment which are the passive reaction to our thoughts.

Perhaps now we can better understand why we experience an elevated sense of self-worth and control over our lives, **real self-esteem**, when we change our eating habits from irrational, that is, excessive or unreasonable dieting or eating based on excessive restraint alternating with rebellion against the deprivation, to healthy, sensible or rational but tasty choices based on our body's physiological needs.

It is not the shape of our body or the weight we have lost, but the **changed, corrected, thinking pattern based on sound reasoning and self-respect that creates the self-esteem.**

If we decide not to judge the validity or appropriateness of our emotional responses, but instead we permit ourselves to be carried along passively — to go with the flow of our feelings — we **give away the sense of control over our life and thus loose the sense of self-regulation and mastery thereafter: whether we are consciously aware of it or not, we voluntarily undermine and gradually destroy our own sense of worthiness.**

As children, we are at first not consciously aware of the fact that there is a range of choices in our thoughts, feelings and behaviors, some choices better than others and some that need to be avoided.

Before we learn to appreciate and use the privilege and power of our free will, we first need to learn or preferably be taught by our caretakers that some of our desires are appropriate and good for us while others are not.

We also need to learn to evaluate our feelings and desires not only in reference to how they affect us, but, also how they affect others around us. Learning that we are entitled to some things and not others, forms the basis of all our future relationships as well as, our own sense of appropriate boundaries and entitlement, that is, our sense of worthiness.

The essential qualities, first of awareness and secondly of discernment or the ability to judge between principled and unprincipled thinking and living form the very structure of our moral fiber and character. These earliest beginnings are much more important and carry more far-reaching consequences than most parents realize.

In his book, *The Psychology of Self-Esteem*, Dr. Brandon gives the example of a child who wants another's toy, really badly, but even though the child senses this is wrong (because he wouldn't want his friend to take his toy), the child overrides this inner sense, this reasonable or rational thinking, and takes the toy anyway. Long after the incident is forgotten, the consequences remain — "that **it is permissible,**

at times, to ignore knowledge and facts in order to indulge a desire. This is the legacy of his theft — this, plus a residue of vague, nameless guilt, the sense of some inner uncleanliness, **the state of a mind learning to distrust itself."***

Applying this reasoning to desires of appetite: we know that eating beyond the feeling of fullness is not good for us. If we eat too much anyway, we erode our self-esteem.

In the future, the child can either change this pattern by choosing not to take what doesn't belong to him, or **"reinforce it by repeated acts of evasion and irrational emotional indulgence,*** which undermine his self-esteem still further."

Such injury to self-esteem results from **any** irrational, emotional indulgence. Thus, willful disobedience in childhood, instigated by immature emotional responses and allowed to go on due to lack of parental discipline, has far-reaching and serious consequences on a child's development of self-worth. A lamentable legacy, it may take the rest of the person's life to correct — **if**, in adulthood, he or she is fortunate enough to discover the cause of their problem:

> *that they betrayed their mind by being allowed to indulge in desires stimulated by feelings which overrode rational thinking based on principles.*

It is truly a shame that:

> *the majority of "people", as adults, suffer from a significant deficit of self-esteem. The senseless tragedy of their lives is that most of them betrayed their mind, not for the sake of gratifying some violent if irrational passion, but for the sake of indulging meaningless or senseless whims that they can no longer remember, for the sake of being free to act on the impulse or spur of the moment, without the responsibility of awareness or thought.*
>
> Nathaniel Brandon

There is no point assigning blame for this lack of teaching to either parents or the school system. The most well-meaning parents may not

---

* bold type added

be aware of the harm they are causing their children by over-indulgence or lack of consistent but loving discipline. The children can not be blamed either as they are totally at the mercy of their caretakers until they are grown up enough to take care of themselves.

However, adults do have the choice to re-educate and re-parent themselves and although it may not be easy and may take some time, the gain of worthiness, empowerment, peace of mind, and happiness, among other positive effects, are well worth the extended effort.

Without the effort of learning how to think rationally and correct any distorted patterns of thinking and feeling, the continued lack of awareness, the refusal to accept complete responsibility for our thoughts and actions and to be disciplined enough to be guided by principled thinking and behaving as outlined in Chapter 8, is an abuse of a uniquely human gift: the gift of free will.

Such abuse has serious consequences in our life resulting from the damage sustained to self-esteem. It causes a feeling of separation from what is good, which results in feelings of physical and emotional dis-ease in various degrees. These can fluctuate from time to time all the way from physical illness and despair to mild irritability, restlessness or dissatisfaction with oneself including one's appearance as well as others, which may lead to dissatisfaction in personal and working relationships. In other words, a life not lived with enjoyment to the full extent of one's potential.

It is unfortunate that often it is not until a major life crisis occurs that we are confronted or forced to deal with these issues.

Our best guide to what is right and what will add to our self-esteem or wrong and will undermine it, is to ask the following:

In reference to ourselves we need to inquire: "is this thought or action going to be beneficial to my health and well-being, or is it going to be detrimental?"

We also need to ask this question when making a decision regarding any cosmetic surgery or treatment. We need to rationally decide whether the benefits of the procedure outweigh the risks, and, whether we are willing to live with the consequences of the risks.

Remember, true self-esteem comes from thinking rationally not running away from situations that are difficult and not basing our decisions on what feels more comfortable and safe.

In reference to others, we need to inquire: "is this the way I would want to be treated myself?"

If it is not, then change it.

This principle applies to all of our thoughts and actions. If we make a commitment and break it; if we speak negatively about someone behind their back, thinking they will not hear us or find out about it; if we borrow any money, however little, and do not repay it, it will **hurt us and only us**.

The other person may not even be aware of what we say, or he may forget that he lent us money. But our mind will not forget; neither will it be fooled by rationalizations, such as, "He was mean to me — I have a right to say mean things about him in return;" or, "She lent me money, but I did other things for her in return — and she can afford it anyway. I don't have as much money as she does."

Likewise, if someone hurts or mistreats us, we do not have to retaliate. In fact, we do not want to retaliate. Retaliation will only hurt us by the same marvelous, built-in boomerang mechanism that will, sooner rather than later, return to affect the person responsible for the dishonest or negative thought or action and may consist of the person responsible simply feeling bad for no obviously apparent reason.

> *He who digs another man a grave will fall into it himself.*
> **Slovak Proverb**

Of course, this also applies to positive thoughts and actions, the fruit of which will also return to their originator.

> *Any person who contributes to prosperity must prosper in turn.*
> **Earl Nightingale**

There is no doubt that rejecting thinking based on reason under the pressure of irrational desires or unethical thinking has disastrous consequences on our life. But, what is even more disastrous is rejecting our mind under the pressure of fear.

*The underlying cause of **all** trouble is fear.*

                                        Emmet Fox

*Fear is a thief who sneaks around inside you, stealing your happiness. A chief danger in fear is that a man **never sees how afraid he really is**. So he lies and bluffs all day, but never deceives his own nature. He shivers over everything but is especially worried that his world might fall apart. This occurs when a close human relationship breaks down, exposing his fakery. Submit fear to the spirit of sanity. Sanity will win. You will win.*

                                    Vernon Howard

Our attitude toward fear and our method of dealing with it is crucial to our psychological and spiritual well-being.

If, when confronted by a fearful situation, we allow the fear to take over and control our consciousness and we run away, the fearful situation and our avoidance of it becomes a reflection of our personal worth. If the fear assumes more importance than the opportunity to show courage and master the fearful situation, and we give up instead of rising to meet the difficulty, the fear becomes our master. Although we may not consciously be aware of it, our subconscious mind registers humiliation and self-doubt, which initiate negative, self-depreciating thoughts that are disempowering and deplete our self-esteem.

Running away from a fearful situation undermines our sense of self-esteem.

Here again, parents have the opportunity to make a major difference to their child's development of strong self-esteem by teaching him or her how to deal with fear.

If your parents did not teach you how to deal with fear, you can learn to deal with it on your own, by asking yourself the following rational questions suggested by Dr. David Viscott:

Why am I afraid?

What is the worst that could happen to me?

What are the chances of the worst taking place?

How do I know? How can I limit my loss?

Can I get out of the situation before the worst happens?

Immediate retreat without first thinking it through is not coping rationally with fear, unless, of course, we are confronted by immediate physical danger, such as a man with a gun or a tiger on the loose. Thinking through the situation and finding a solution is coping rationally. Further, as we grow from childhood to adulthood, fear becomes masked in many different ways.

Fear is often disguised as logical and rational reasons why something cannot be done. Sometimes it comes disguised as a feeling that other people are stopping you. There are many ways to disguise fear — blame it on others, refuse to take responsibility, decide you can't do it anyway so why try, get angry and quit, and many others. What ways do you cover up fear?

Sanaya Roman

Overcoming fearful situations is a source of self-esteem.

Overcoming fear and building self-esteem is based on a choice: to think or not to think with wisdom and clarity.

This may sound like a simple task and in fact it is, until we find ourselves in a situation where the trigger button for our habitual distorted thinking is pushed either intentionally or unintentionally. Unless we have previously prepared ourselves to respond automatically, like a professional athlete responds to the sound of the starter pistol, with rational thinking without any distortion, the speed with which our thinking occurs driven by the force of habit will quickly launch us on the negative, downhill path of self-depreciation and self-destruction.

To break a habit of distorted thinking, especially if there are several, requires extra effort, the most important of which is the assumption of personal responsibility.

This is particularly important when making any decisions regarding our body or personal well-being.

For example, if we undergo a cosmetic procedure to please some-one else and thereby abandon or neglect the responsibility we have to ourselves and we do not like the result or worse still, if something goes wrong and we are scarred, we will likely feel alienated and resentful toward ourselves, the world, and everyone in it — especially the peo-ple we mistakenly hold responsible for our own abdication of self-responsibility.

Our self-esteem is not dependent on particular successes or fail-ures, since these may involve factors that are outside our conscious control, such as the participation of other people. It would be unwise and in fact dangerous to do so under these circumstances as we have limited control over what other people do. What is required of us is to remain open to honest evaluation based on reality and to use our mind to our fullest ability at all times and under all circumstances.

Self-esteem requires continued effort every day for the rest of our lives. Just as we need to breathe, so we need to use our mind con-structively and productively to maintain our self-esteem. In fact, the greater the challenges we seek **and overcome**, the greater the growth of our self-esteem.

In summary, as Dr. Brandon notes:

> ...an individual who develops healthily, derives intense pleasure and pride from the work of his mind, and from the achievements which that work makes possible. Feeling confident of his ability to deal with the facts of reality, he will want a chal-lenging, effortful, **creative** existence.
>
> Creativeness will be his highest love, whatever his level of intelligence.
>
> The principle that distinguishes the basic moti-vation of a man of self-esteem from that of a man of pseudo self-esteem, is the principle of **motivation**

*by love versus **motivation by fear**. Love of self and of existence — versus the fear that one's self is unfit for existence. Motivation by **confidence** — versus motivation by terror.*

*To the extent that a man lacks self-esteem, he lives **negatively** and **defensively**. When he chooses his particular values and goals, his primary motive is, not to afford himself a positive enjoyment but to defend himself against anxiety, against painful feelings of inadequacy, self-doubt and guilt."*

Acting defensively may temporarily or partly ward off the threat of exposing publicly what we are so afraid of and anxious to cover up, but it does not protect us from ourselves. Our subconscious mind can not be deceived. It knows the truth regardless of the defenses and excuses which we consciously create.

The best way to deal with our subconscious mind and the only way to gain peace and achieve maximum benefit is to become aware of our feelings and their origin in our thinking as clearly and honestly as we can; then accept the responsibility for them, and after evaluating their benefit to us and others around us make a decision based on reason and ethical guidelines, to change what is not beneficial. This, however, requires a **willingness** to change and grow.

CHAPTER

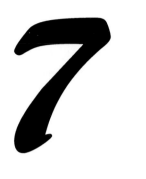

WILLINGNESS TO GROW BEAUTIFUL

ACCEPT THE CHALLENGE TO LEARN AND GROW

Once we have decided to accept the challenge, we need to look at our problems as lessons from which to learn and grow. We need to be serious students of what life has to offer.

> *The wise man is glad to be instructed, but a self-sufficient fool falls flat on his face.*
>
> **Proverbs 10:8**

> *The intelligent man is always open to new ideas. In fact, he looks for them.*
>
> **Proverbs 18:15**

It is crucial that we **learn** from any painful or unpleasant experiences and **change our thinking** accordingly. If we don't do this, we will continue to be confronted by these same problems and painful feelings, just disguised as different problems, in different situations.

It is very important, however, that while we learn from negative thoughts and experiences, we do so with kindness and compassion.

*We must **learn to be kind to our minds**. Let's*

*not hate ourselves for having negative thoughts. We can think of our thoughts as **building** us up rather than **beating** us up. We don't have to blame ourselves for negative experiences. We can learn from these experiences. Being kind to ourselves means to stop all blame, all guilt, all punishment, and all pain.*

Louise L. Hay

In this regard, relationships with people present some of the most valuable opportunities for growth.

*You may think that the best friends are those who never challenge you, who never make you want to close your heart, and yet if you are with people who never challenge you to remain open and loving, you are not truly connecting with them in your heart. The heart always deals with issues of trusting, opening and reaching new levels of acceptance and understanding of others. **You learn to love by putting yourself in situations that challenge you to be loving.***

Sanaya Roman

Your enemies are those who approve of your wrong behavior, and your friends are those who disapprove, and that is all there is to it.

Here is how to be your own best friend.

Know that the lies you tell yourself are the same lies you are eager to hear from others. Deceitfully believing that you are doing what is best for yourself, you cling to those who agree with your fakery. You think they are your true friends when they are really traitors who scorn you enough to bind you to your sad act. A woman said, "He was the only man who loved me enough to quietly tell me I was

---

* bold type added

all wrong." Remember this.

Vernon Howard

The key here is straightforwardness. Anyone who in the name of *concern* for us, *trying* to be helpful talks behind our back and *magnifies* problems by indulging in gossip, yet is all smiles and reassurances to our face, is not a friend. Friends will tell us what they think to our face, even if what they have to say may be painful. Behind our back, they will defend us.

True friends will **BE** helpful, not just claim to be helpful. They will confront us directly and *offer a solution* to our problem.

However, people with a negative perspective are most likely in trouble themselves and cannot help us out anyway, no matter how much they intend to do so. As the blind cannot lead the blind, so destructive negativity leads only to more negativity and destruction.

We might well reflect on the difference between constructive and destructive criticism.

Constructive criticism identifies problems and solves them with solutions. It uses crises to build strength.

> *Don't refuse to accept criticism; get all the help you can.*
> **Proverbs 23:12**

> *Anyone willing to be corrected is on the pathway to life. Anyone refusing has lost his chance.*
> **Proverbs 13:18**

Destructive criticism magnifies the problem by assigning blame without offering or wanting solutions. Its purpose is to use crises as character assassinations.

> *Everything that happens to you is your teacher. The secret is to learn to sit at the feet of your own life and be taught by it.*

> *Everything that happens is either a blessing which is also a lesson, or a lesson which is also a blessing.*
> **Polly Berrien Berends**

All criticism is unpleasant. However, it is detrimental to our well-being to reject all criticism as undesirable, judgmental and unloving. Learn to tell the difference. To avoid it altogether, be your own teacher. Ask yourself what lessons you can learn from any unpleasant feelings you are experiencing.

For example, in response to a criticism from your boss, you can say to yourself, "My boss cares about the quality of the work we do. I have a chance to learn something here" and then proceed to learn all you can. Rather than becoming angry, defensive, and vindictive, listen to his or her point of view then try to work out how you can best meet his or her needs and expectations. By responding with empathy and understanding you will not only ensure that your boss will be satisfied with how you handled the complaint but you will end up feeling more confident and better about yourself.

> *Light a candle, rather than complain about the darkness.*
> **Chinese Proverb**

Reason with yourself and try to understand the causes of every situation where painful feelings overwhelm you. Do not condemn yourself or feel guilty about the painful or negative feelings. Just observe their passage through your own consciousness from a distance as though you were watching someone else and then return to your centered, and constructively positive position as soon as possible.

> *The more you understand what you are learning from a situation, the more rapidly you can leave it.*
> **Sanaya Roman**

MISTAKES

Learning from mistakes deserves a special mention, since mistakes are our greatest teachers.

If you make a mistake, admit it and learn from it as quickly as possible. Then move on, determined not to make the same mistake again.

> *Don't be afraid to fail. Don't waste energy on trying to cover up failure. Learn from your failures*

and go on to the next challenge. It's O.K. to fail. If you're not failing, you're not growing.

H. Stanley Judd

Not many people are willing to give failure a second opportunity. They fail once and it's all over. The bitter pill of failure...is often more than most people can handle....If you're willing to accept failure and learn from it, if you're willing to consider failure as a blessing in disguise and bounce back, you've got the potential of harnessing one of the most powerful success forces.

Joseph Sugarman

ADMITTING TO MISTAKES IS A SOURCE OF GREAT INTERNAL STRENGTH

We can not predict or control all external circumstances or other people's actions or reactions. For this reason and because we are not infallible, there is always a potential for mistakes to occur.

While we cannot control other people, we can control ourselves. Mistakes give us the opportunity to learn about ourselves. When we learn about ourselves, we acquire awareness and understanding which guide us toward changing ourselves for the better. By being able to change our response, we can avoid a particular mistake in the future. This gives us power not only to avoid the same mistakes but also their consequences on our life.

Additionally, if we thus learn to rely on ourselves to resolve problems, we will not feel compelled to use food as a comfort nor will we indulge other compulsions that temporarily dampen the pain of not taking responsibility for our actions and our lives. Such compulsive behavior will only add to our poor self-image, and it is poor self-image that

...is the magnifying glass that can transform a trivial mistake or an imperfection into an overwhelming symbol of personal defeat.

David Burns

It would be wonderful if, at the perfect moment, when everything is going well and we are happy, we could stop the changes in our life and continue living in that constant bliss. Apart from being unrealistic, such an existence would eventually result in boredom.

Some people overcome overwhelming odds, while others whose lives are seemingly perfect are unhappy. The difference is attitude. Your attitude determines whether you perceive a situation as an exciting challenge or as a stressful problem. A stepping stone or a stumbling block.

> *We do not see things as they are. We see them as we are.*
>
> **The Talmud**

So, if you haven't already, open yourself to a new way of thinking and feeling. You have the power to change. Take control of your life and you have found the secret to happiness and a longer and healthier life.

> *It is not easy to find happiness in ourselves, and it is not possible to find it elsewhere.*
>
> **Agnes Repplier**

CHAPTER

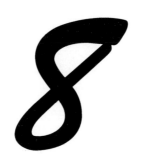

BELIEVING BEAUTIFUL

REVIEW YOUR BELIEF SYSTEM

Even when we *want* to eliminate distorted thinking patterns, the process will not occur overnight. It may take some time, depending on the degree of motivation, self-awareness, and our belief system. In fact, in addition to changing distorted thinking patterns, it is crucial to examine and review our belief system from time to time. For if our beliefs are faulty, our thinking will be also.

This is especially important if destructive thoughts continue to appear. In such a case, try to determine what in your belief system could be causing the distorted thinking patterns. Be totally honest with yourself. Are you thinking from a self-centered position that is distorting your view of the reality of any situation? Does your real intent match what you have said or how you have acted?

In general, it is helpful to determine what is important to you. What is the ideal way you would like to be. Which qualities of character do you most value and admire. Take the time to evaluate what you want out of life. Be specific. There is no road to success but through a clear, strong purpose. What is your mission in life? Write down exactly what you want and what you want to change. Then gently but firmly claim what you want by seeing yourself as already having achieved it.

> *Commit yourself to a dream. You affirm you are*
> *created in the image of God, that you have latent*
> *talent and abilities, that you deserve to succeed as*
> *much as anybody else, and after you begin to*
> *believe that somehow, some way, somewhere,*
> *sometime, through someone you can make it.*
>
> *When you are inspired with a dream, God has*
> *hit the ball into your court. Now you have to hit it*
> *back with commitment.*
>
> **Robert Schuller**

Do not be impatient, disbelieving, or worried about how the fulfillment of your dreams will come about. Your subconscious mind will do the job for you once it has accepted the idea of having or being whatever you want. Its power is such that it will automatically direct your actions toward fulfillment.

Be sure to choose your direction or wishes wisely. After you get what you thought you wanted, you may find that it was not what you wanted at all. Purely materialistic desires do not lead to happiness or contentment.

As Thomas Crum points out in *The Magic of Conflict*, nearly all concrete wishes (whether for material possessions or a face lift or a slimmer waist) spring from the desire for a quality of being or ideal, such as love, respect, or understanding. It is easy to fall into the trap of believing that "if I were only prettier, smarter or richer, I would have something more to offer, and my loved ones would love me, respect me or need me more."

The greatest and most beneficial realization is that when we learn to love ourselves more – which is the essence of the real need behind our wishes — then our loved ones will love us more without us changing anything.

> *Treasure the love you receive above all. It will*
> *survive long after your gold and good health have*
> *vanished .*
>
> **Og Mandino**

Quality life is built on solid principles of right living, such as truth, honesty, and intelligent love – that is, love guided by wisdom, compassion and empathy (not just sentimental feelings). Loyalty, strength and undaunted, self-disciplined perseverance or will power are necessary if we are to abide by these principles on a daily basis. Even if, and especially when the going gets tough and it would be easier not to do so, to just give up – and do what "feels" better or requires less effort.

God did not give us a spirit of timidity, but a
spirit of power, of love and of self-discipline.

2 Timothy 1:7

The reward is built in: when we live and work in alignment with these principles we experience inner joy and satisfaction, we feel inherently uplifted when goodness and justice triumph over their opposites. However, it is best to live by these principles not because they are rewarded but because right living allows the inner imperative, the true nature of our being to surface and come to light for all the world to see. There is an inner law in the very depths of our being that directs us to think and do what is right. The consequence of not obeying this law is discontent, unhappiness, dis-ease and disharmony in our life.

All spiritual teachings have as their basis the same clear guidelines of correct thinking or code of conduct. It does not matter what religion you practice or whether you practice any at all. All spiritual teaching and all civilized societies are founded on the basics set out by the Ten Commandments.

The general and basic premise that makes these guidelines universally applicable is the belief in the *one* unifying benevolent presence shared by all creation. That is, God. Whatever we believe, the mystery of life is beyond our comprehension, but its presence cannot be denied.

The following are ten basic, universally accepted guidelines of correct conduct based on the Ten Commandments. These are universal truths which have withstood the test of time and form the foundation of both East and West spiritual teachings.*

I **Devotion**. This is a means of expressing and living the belief in

---

* as outlined by John Novak in his book, *How to Meditate.*

the one power of God who unifies all of life. It is the opening of our heart to encompass principles of value rather than material objects. In practical terms, this means doing everything with interested involvement, for the sake of doing it, especially for the sake of doing good, not for the material or emotional rewards. The reward of devotion is perfect happiness, serenity and unlimited success in all endeavors.

II **Non-Violence**. This is an attitude of good will to all, or, at least, one of not harming any other creature. It includes not taking advantage of others in any way whatever — for example, not boosting the ego by demeaning others or withholding credit where it is due. As we all have experienced, hidden deep in the recesses of our fallible subconscious *human* mind, are such tendencies as self-righteousness, fault-finding, hostility, and violence. On the other hand, the reward of thoughts of good will is peace and harmony and consequently good physical health.

III **Non-Lying**. This means not only *not saying* anything that is untruthful but also being completely honest with ourselves at all times. Without such complete honesty, we may perceive falsely and rationalize that the only *truth* is what we believe it to be from our limited, ego-conscious point of view. The reward of honesty is personal power: that is, whatever good we think and pray for will come to pass.

IV **Non-Stealing**. Apart from the obvious, this includes more subtle thoughts and ways of not taking what doesn't belong to us. For example, not taking credit for others' work or not taking up time or even affection and support from someone unless it has been freely offered. The reward is the automatic attraction of wealth when it is needed.

V **Non-Sensuality**. This is the practice of self-control. In other words, the rational reasoning thinking process that overrides feelings instigated by the senses (what feels good at the time), in favor of the greatest good of the individual and others. Allowing ourselves to be directed to think and act by feelings alone is like being tossed in a small boat on the high seas. Tremendous energy is spent just staying afloat and preventing the drowning of our human consciousness in any one feeling. The strength that comes as a result of staying anchored by reason and "learning not to waste our energy through the senses is tremendous mental and spiritual vitality."

VI **Non-Greed**. Greed stems from some level of insecurity, and as we mature spiritually, we develop a deep faith in God. Non-greed also includes transcending, by our firm faith, more subtle insecurities such as the craving for others' constant approval or compliments. The reward is a lack of fear and acquisition of faith and a clear vision of our past, present and future.

VII **Cleanliness**. This is an externalization of inner order and purity. Its reward "is a divine indifference to things related to the body." This does not mean neglect. On the contrary, it means a balanced concern and care, but not to the point of obsession. The reward is self-appreciation and clear vision. How much we appreciate ourselves is a measure of how valuable and worthy we feel. This in turn directly contributes to our self-esteem and personal effectiveness in taking command over our life and destiny. Clear vision gives us the ability to avoid making mistakes.

Thus, something as mundane and at first glance seemingly unimportant, as clean and tidy surroundings is a reflection of the state of our mind and attitude toward ourselves and others with profound and far-reaching effects on our whole life.

VIII **Contentment**. This means to be accepting and appreciative of life in general. To go with the flow but not to the point of apathy or laziness. It means to be in command of the calm strength to both accept things as they are and also to change certain of those same things as needed. Contentment reflects an attitude of gratitude. If we are grateful for what life has to offer, we are more likely to be appreciative or at least accepting of the ups and downs. The reward of contentment is patience, peace of mind, mastery of any work or life situation, satisfaction and happiness experienced at all times.

IX **Austerity**. This combines mastering ourselves through the self-disciplined application of reason and "the strength of determination" to do what reason and faith guide us to do. It means to gain understanding over our own lack of understanding or misguided thoughts. The reward is special gifts "that come with perfection of this virtue," such as healing of self and others.

X **Self-Study**. This means self-awareness by honest introspection. This does not mean being self-critical in a negative sense or beating ourselves over the head if we perceive imperfections. It means to simply see ourselves completely as we are, in an objective, detached manner. The reward of introspection is progress on the spiritual path. "Without introspection, it is next to impossible to progress on the spiritual path." In fact the translation of the Hebrew word for prayer is self-analysis. Our prayers are answered as a result of honest and constructive self-awareness and change of our consciousness for the better, in line with these principles.

Abiding by these principles is the high road of life. It initially appears to be the more difficult way to go but in the long run is the only way that leads to a quality life.

> In the main stream of life two currents, especially, may be observed. One is toward an expansion of awareness. The other is a sinking back into sleep and unawareness, a shutting out of reality, a longing for death. Positive and negative — in all of us, both of these trends may be observed.

> To the extent that we draw the world to us, by an attitude of willingness, appreciation, kindness, joy, we express the positive current. When, by unwillingness, a critical attitude, selfishness, unkindness, grief, we push the world away from us, excluding it from our circle of awareness, we express the negative current.

> ...our virtues and vices are not really we, ourselves. They are reflections, only, of the plane of consciousness on which we live. As that plane changes, the traits of our personality change also.

>   J. Donald Walters
>   (Kriyananda)

Viewed from this perspective of understanding, the instructions given to us by the true spiritual teachers, the enlightened ones, are very practical.

If, however, we do not share their understanding, we may miss out on the valuable instruction that these teachings provide for our everyday life.

THE REWARD OF INNER BEAUTY

This world is a school — that and nothing more; and provided you learn your lesson, nothing else matters. It does not really matter whether you are rich or poor, cultured or simple, a king or a scavenger. These are only the roles that men enact on the stage of life. **How the role is acted is what matters.** * *The two supreme lessons set for this school are the lesson of* **(seeing the presence of something beneficial in every situation),** * *and the lesson of the* **power of thought.** * *Every negative or difficult thing that enters into our life marks our inability to realize (the presence of something beneficial),* * *and it is therefore but the signal for another step to be made. Make that step in spiritual (creative),* * *understanding, and never again throughout eternity will that particular task have to be done.*

The power of thought is the second great lesson that we have to master....

Emmet Fox

It would be nice if our parents or the school system taught us these principal purposes of life and how to achieve them in our childhood, when we are more receptive, more able to grasp new concepts.

Some of us are fortunate to have had parents who did teach us. All parents do the best they know how, at the time. They, too, are children, all but grown up, whose parents did the best they knew how.

What we are taught and what we find out for ourselves about dealing with life is like a boat, a raft with which we travel on the ocean of life, on our own, once we grow up.

Some children are helped to build ocean liners for their travel, others canoes, and still others are thrown without anything into shark-

* bold type and words in parentheses added

infested waters.

This is the legacy of childhood and parenting, about which we can do nothing. The past is done and gone forever.

However, as adults, we can do something now, in the present. If we do not like the way we are coping with life, or if we do not like the quality of our life, we can choose to see how we are facing the world and then choose to change it as needed to achieve the highest quality of life, to which all of us have equal access and which all of us deserve.

Once we become aware and determined to do so, we can rebuild the boat in which we are now travelling — by choosing to base our thinking on the principles of truth, honesty, rational, positive, intuitive and wise thinking, which can change the experience of our ocean travels now and in the future.

HAPPY SAILING!!

PART TWO

EXTERNAL BEAUTY

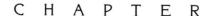

C H A P T E R

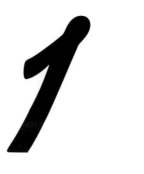

UNDERSTANDING OUR SKIN

Knowing about the structure and function of our skin will help us understand what is and isn't good for it, and why.

The skin is the largest organ in our body. It is ⅟₄₈ to ⅕ of an inch (0.5 mm to 5.0 mm) thick and covers an area of about 5 to 6.5 square feet (1.5 to 2 square meters).

It's primary function is to protect the body by forming a barrier against environmental stresses such as cold, heat, ultraviolet light, germs and even chemical or mechanical injury.

Skin is composed of three layers. The two outer layers are firmly attached to one another: the outer-most layer is the epidermis; and the inner is the dermis. Beneath these two layers is the fatty layer called the subcutaneous tissue, which acts as an insulator, calorie reserve and shock absorber.

THE STRUCTURE OF SKIN

The Epidermis

The epidermis is made up of multiple cell layers. The bottom layer at the base of the epidermis is the regenerative or basal zone. Cells in this single layer, called basal cells, are constantly dividing, *mostly during sleep.*

As new cells form in the basal layer, they are pushed upward towards the surface of the skin by younger cells beneath and eventually become flattened. They manufacture keratin protein and die on their way to the surface.

The surface layer of the epidermis is made up of old dry cells that are continually lost in the form of microscopic flakes. It takes about one month for the epidermis in human skin to completely renew itself.

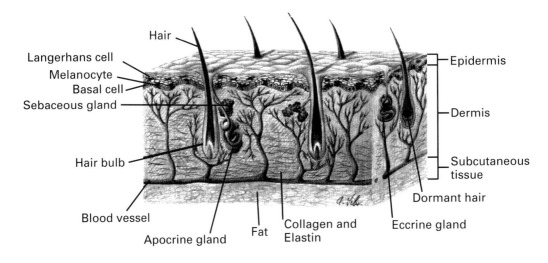

Hair

Langerhans cell
Melanocyte
Basal cell
Sebaceous gland

Epidermis

Dermis

Hair bulb

Subcutaneous tissue

Dormant hair

Blood vessel

Apocrine gland   Fat   Collagen and Elastin   Eccrine gland

A CROSS-SECTION OF THE SKIN

Keratin is a protein and is the main component of the outer cell layers. It is almost waterproof. This is what makes it possible to take a bath in fresh water without the body becoming swollen with water, or in salt water without shrinking.

The entire body can, therefore, be conceptualized as being encased within a husk. This husk or shield has a protective function, acting as a barrier to water and other substances and organisms. Its thickness is related to the mechanical forces encountered as well as its location on the body. Pressure and friction tend to increase its thickness as does sun bathing. It is, therefore, thickest on the palms and soles of the feet and areas of the body with the most severe sun damage.

However, the epidermis is not completely impervious. Many chemicals can be absorbed through it. Be careful, then, to avoid direct contact with chemicals, insecticides, solvents and other toxic materials like paints and kerosene. Furthermore, if the keratin layer becomes too wet or water-logged from prolonged bathing, it will lose some of its protective function and become more permeable to water and other substances. Over time, this results in considerable loss of water and dry skin. In addition, if the protective fatty-film surface, that the skin normally produces, is removed with soap and water or degreasing agents such as alcohol, there will be even more water loss.

The surface fatty-film consists of two types of oils: those produced by the epidermis, and those manufactured in the dermis by sebaceous glands. Those made by the sebaceous glands are made up of fatty substances that are thicker than those produced by the epidermis, and are called sebum.

The function of the surface oils is to help skin retain moisture and to lubricate its surface. They make the surface of the skin acidic rather than neutral or alkaline. The acidity may have some anti-bacterial functions.

The epidermis also contains pigment cells called melanocytes which are situated in the bottom layer and produce a brown or red pigment called melanin. Melanin protects skin from sunlight by absorbing some of the harmful ultraviolet (UV) rays. However, in fair or untanned skin, not enough melanin may be present to result in any significant protection.

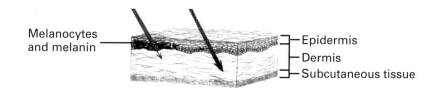

HOW UV LIGHT PENETRATES THE SKIN

Only a small amount of UV light is required for the epidermis to produce vitamin D. For people with fair complexions, this may be as little as fifteen minutes once or twice a week. More than this can be harmful by causing sunburn and, after many years of exposure, causing skin cancers.

Vitamin D is essential for the maintenance of normal bone structure, bone growth and repair. In particular, it is needed for the absorption of calcium from the intestine. Calcium is an important mineral for building strong bones. The active part of vitamin D is made in the skin by the action of sunlight, and in the kidneys.

Finally, the epidermis also serves an important function in our immune system. Immune cells, called Langerhans cells, act as police: by recognizing germs and other foreign substances, they notify other parts of our immune system to mount an appropriate response to reject any intruder such as harmful chemicals. These cells may be damaged by exposure to even small amounts of UV light.

The exact mechanism by which UV light causes skin cancer is not yet known. It is known that UV light causes direct damage to the genetic content of skin cells leading to mutations or "mis-spelled" genes. If enough mis-spelling occurs, the cell becomes cancerous. In the presence of a healthy immune system, such faulty cells would normally be rejected.

Under some circumstances, however, such rejection may not be beneficial. For example, following severe or prolonged exposure of a fair-skinned individual to UV light, when large numbers of skin cells may suffer direct damage. If, under these circumstances, these damaged cells were all rejected at the same time shortly after exposure, the survival of the individual may be at risk due to infection and loss of essential body fluids through the ulcerated skin where the sun-damaged skin cells were rejected.

Under these circumstances, suppression of the immune system would prevent the immediate loss of the sun-damaged skin cells and could therefore be considered of survival value to the excessively sunburnt individual with fair skin. UV light does, in fact, also damage skin immune cells. In the absence of these cells (Langerhans cells), the mis-spelled epidermal cells will be not only, not rejected but actively supported by the immune system. This active suppression of the immune defense mechanism will enable the cancerous cells to grow instead of being rejected, thus preventing the more immediate threat to survival.

Fortunately, it takes many years for such sun-induced skin cancers to grow to a size large enough to become noticeable and even longer to grow large enough to be dangerous. They are also easily treated and unless allowed to grow to a large size, rarely result in serious problems. The active suppression of immune rejection of sun-damaged skin, for example after a severe sunburn, would therefore seem to be beneficial in the short term, promoting the survival of an individual whose skin burns easily in a sunny, hot climate.

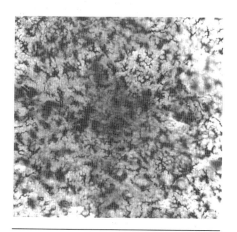

Langerhans cells in the epidermis of a person with fair skin before exposure to ultraviolet light.

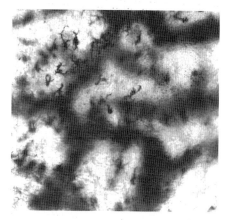

Langerhans cells in the same person after exposure to 15 minutes of simulated sunlight on 3 consecutive days.

Thus, the UV light-induced, temporary immune suppression and the consequent acceptance of the damaged skin cells could be viewed as a protective survival mechanism.

Melanoma, on the other hand, is a cancer of pigment cells and spreads easily to other organs in the body. Early removal is essential and will usually result in cure. If left to grow, melanoma is deadly.

Because the epidermis has no blood vessels, it receives nutrition from fluid that passes from the dermis into spaces between the cells in the epidermis. Improving blood flow in the dermis by exercise and massage can be beneficial for nutrition of the epidermis. Gentle facials are helpful in this regard for maintaining a healthy, glowing complexion.

The Dermis

The dermis comprises the middle layer and provides the skin with much of its strength and elasticity. Elasticity refers to the ability of skin to be stretched and then to return to its original shape. The dermis contains the blood vessels, lymph drainage channels and nerve endings that supply the epidermis, as well as hair, sweat and oil glands.

The dermis is composed of a dense network of collagen and elastin fibers. Both collagen and elastin fibers are made of protein. The difference between them is that the main function of collagen is to provide strength and support and elastin to provide the ability to stretch and recoil.

The great majority of dermal connective tissues are composed of collagen. Only 1% of the total is composed of elastin.

The dermis interlocks with the epidermis in a series of ridges and valleys. This interlocking is mechanically advantageous because it allows the skin to be stretched, pulled or squeezed without the top two layers separating. When mechanical demands such as stretching and pulling are slight, for example on the face and trunk, there are few, low and irregular ridges. Where the demands are greater, for example around joints, there is more interlocking.

The Basement Membrane

Lining the ridges of the dermis is a thin membrane that separates the dermis and epidermis. It is known as the basement membrane. This structure serves as a filter. It prevents large molecules (particles) such as those composing chemicals and germs, from passing between the two layers.

Subcutaneous Tissue

Beneath the dermis is the subcutaneous tissue. It is made up of a loose network of fibers interspersed between lobules or deposits of fat. This tissue is often considered part of the skin because it blends into the dermis. In some places, such as the face and neck, there is little or no subcutaneous tissue. In these places, the muscle fibers end directly in the dermis, which facilitates facial movements.

The density and arrangement of the subcutaneous layer help to determine the mobility of skin, which can be considerable in most places, except on the palms and soles. In these sites, subcutaneous tissue is more taut than it is elsewhere.

Lymphatic Channels

Lymphatics are vessels that collect fluid called lymph fluid, which drains from spaces between skin cells. This liquid surrounds cells and contains nutrients delivered to cells by blood vessels, as well as waste substances released by the skin and other cells.

Lymphatic channels are easily blocked by outside pressure or lack of the usual activity of underlying muscles, which normally helps to move lymph fluid through these thin-walled vessels. Excess accumulation of lymph fluid may lead to swelling, called edema. Both exercise and massage will help lymph fluid drain.

IN AND AROUND THE SKIN

Sebaceous Or Oil Glands

Sebaceous glands are situated in the dermis and are found almost everywhere on the body except the palms and soles. They produce an oily substance called sebum, which is discharged into the hair canal and forms a protective coating on the surface of the skin. Sebum is constantly produced, as the excess is continuously lost from the surface.

High temperatures may increase the flow of previously formed sebum to the surface, which is why in hot weather your skin may appear oilier. Using soap and water as you would for hygiene has little effect on this film-like barrier. However, excessive washing and use of harsh soaps and solvents will dissolve this layer and reduce its effectiveness as a barrier for the epidermis. Appropriate and specifically designed moisturizing creams can replenish the protective surface film and thus restore the barrier function (see Chapter 6).

Sebaceous glands are primarily influenced by sex hormones, which is why they change size at different times in life. Before puberty, for example, the sebaceous glands are quite small. One of the earliest signs of puberty may be their enlargement. After puberty, the glands remain stable in size until menopause when they begin to decrease in size and activity. In men, oil gland size and level of activity is maintained until about seventy years of age.

Sweat Glands

There are two types of sweat glands called the eccrine and apocrine glands. Both are located in the dermis or underlying fat layer. The apocrine glands are generally deeper than the eccrine glands.

Sweat glands play an important role in heat regulation by producing sweat which evaporates from the surface of skin. This uses up and takes away heat from the sweating skin. Eccrine glands are found on all body surfaces and are particularly numerous on the palms, soles and forehead.

Apocrine glands are fewer in number and found mostly in the skin of the armpits, genitals, abdomen, face, scalp, ear canals and breast nipples. They secrete an oily fluid which contains protein, carbohydrate and ammonia. The secretion may be under the influence of adrenaline as well as some nerve endings. Apocrine glands lack their own canal. Instead, they discharge their contents into the hair canal where it can be mixed with sebaceous secretions.

Hair

Hair is commonly associated with sebaceous glands which discharge their oily contents onto the surface of skin by way of hair canals.

Most of the hair on our body is fine in texture and light in color. Coarser hair is found on the scalp, beard area, under the arms and on the genitals. These coarser hairs may have roots that extend all the way to the subcutaneous layer.

The texture of our hair, its density and rate of growth, vary in different body sites. Sex, age and race also influence the amount of hair we have, its shape, distribution and color.

Baldness and greying of hair, are two of the most obvious changes due to both aging and levels of sex hormones.

Baldness can affect men and women and will follow a similar pattern; hair slowly regresses from the crown of the head and then from the frontal hair-line. One paradox of nature is that when hormone levels in men are at their maximum, scalp hair may be lost while hair on the chest, beard, brows, nostrils and ear canals, is being stimulated to grow!

Hereditary factors influence the onset, degree, rate and pattern of hair loss.

Baldness in women will typically begin later in life and is less severe than in men. If excess balding occurs in young women, it may be due to an over-production of male hormones possibly from an ovarian or adrenal gland tumor, and should be investigated.

Our hair is not constantly growing. At any time, as many as 15-20 percent of scalp hair may be resting. During pregnancy, as many as 30 percent of scalp hairs may be in the dormant stage. Three months after delivery, this may result in temporarily greater hair loss than usual. When the dormant hair bulbs become active again, they usually re-grow new hair.

Physical and psychological stress can also have similar effects on growing hair, causing it to become dormant, followed by a temporary increase in hair loss.

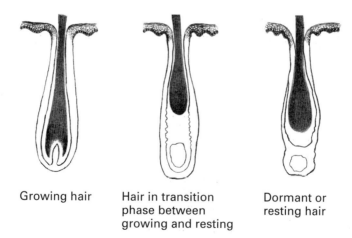

Growing hair   Hair in transition phase between growing and resting   Dormant or resting hair

A CROSS-SECTION OF THE SKIN SHOWING HAIR AT DIFFERENT STAGES

Nails

Nails are found only in humans and other primates. They are specialized structures of the skin and consist of a hard plate which grows on top of a soft bed of blood vessels.

Nails help protect the sensitive finger tips as well as assist in picking up small objects. Unlike our hair, nails grow continuously throughout life.

Although there is considerable individual variation, fingernails grow faster than toenails — at the rate of approximately $\frac{1}{250}$ of an inch (0.1 mm) per day. The fingernails on our dominant hand grow faster than those on our opposite hand. So do the nails on our longest fingers. The peak rates of growth occur during our twenties and thirties, with pregnancy, and in the summer months.

Poor nutrition and illness can slow nail growth.

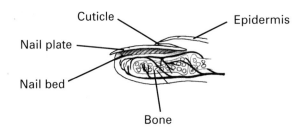

A CROSS-SECTION OF THE FINGER TIP

THE FUNCTIONS OF SKIN

Protection

The primary function of skin is to protect our body from environmental hazards including mechanical injury, ultraviolet light, germs and chemicals. It prevents us from dehydrating or absorbing too much water.

Heat Regulation And Excretion Of Waste Substances

Heat regulation is one of the functions of skin. Sweating acts as a cooling mechanism, as well as a means of ridding the body of undesirable substances.

The blood vessels in the dermis enlarge when the temperature outside is too hot. This brings blood closer to the surface of the skin which allows body heat to escape, and the body is cooled. If the outside temperature is cold, these blood vessels contract and reduce the amount of heat lost and so keep the body warm. Prolonged constriction from severe exposure to cold can result in chilblains or frostbite.

Sensation

All over the body, skin functions as a sensory organ. Nerve endings, responsible for picking up stimuli that evoke various types of sensation including touch, pressure, heat, cold and pain, are found in varying numbers at different body sites. For example, there are more nerve endings on fingers and lips but few on the back. Skin, therefore, plays an essential role in helping people adjust to the environment.

SKIN COLOR

How It Changes

Skin color depends on many factors, including blood flow and the presence of two skin pigments: carotene and melanin. Carotene is the natural food coloring found in yellow or red fruit and vegetables. The tanning pigment melanin, gives skin a brown tone. The amount of pigment present varies greatly and is what makes skin colors range from light tan to dark brown or black. Our skin color is influenced by genetic, environmental and hormonal factors.

Variations in skin color are also due to the amount of blood in the dermal vessels. For example, when someone with fair, white skin is hot, the amount of blood flowing through the blood vessels of the skin is great, which causes skin to look pink to red. On the other hand, when we are cold, blood flows more slowly through the skin and more oxygen is removed by the tissues. Blood that is carrying less oxygen will be darker in color and can even appear to have a bluish tone.

When a person is in shock, the blood vessels to the skin become severely constricted and most of the blood is directed to more vital parts of the body like the heart and brain. The resulting skin color is mostly white or lighter shades of brown to black, unless the carotene content of skin is high. In this case, skin may have a yellow or orange tone.

CHAPTER

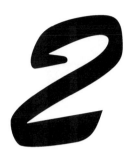

HOW SKIN AGES

How quickly and why skin ages depends on many factors. Genetics, general wear and tear, and environmental stresses are the main culprits. There is no doubt that sun exposure is the single most important environmental factor responsible for accelerating the aging of skin.

Taking care of our skin and avoiding or at least reducing environmental stresses will help us maintain a healthy, youthful complexion for many more years than otherwise expected. However, it is unavoidable that eventually the effects of time, everyday wear and tear, and genetic programming will become apparent.

GENETIC HERITAGE

How Genes Affect Our Skin

The rate at which our skin ages is affected by our genetic endowment as well as how well we care for our skin. Generally, people of Celtic or Scandinavian descent with fair complexions will tend to develop fine, superficial wrinkles more quickly than those with darker complexions. People with dark complexions may develop fewer but deeper facial lines.

Fair skin is less protected and more easily damaged by exposure to sunlight than dark skin. People with fair skin who frequently expose their skin to the sun, will age more quickly than those who protect their skin or those who have naturally dark complexions.

Unfortunately, there is nothing we can do about our genetic heritage, but we can make the best of it by following the common sense rules of nutrition, relaxation, exercise and skin care outlined in the following chapters.

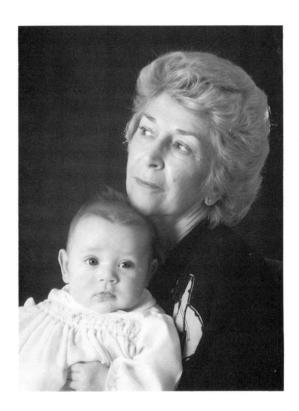

THE EFFECTS OF TIME
How Growing Older Affects Our Skin

As we grow older our body, including our skin, will start to age. The exact mechanism of aging is not yet clearly understood. The biologic clock starts ticking from the time we are born. Eventually, our skin will succumb to the following changes:

- The growth and the repair of tissues slow down, causing all layers of skin to become thinner, less pliable and more easily damaged by everyday stresses.

- Loss of the fatty tissues in the deeper skin layers results in the skin sagging in deeper folds, and being less resistant to cold.

- A decrease in collagen and elastin fibers allows the skin to become lax and lose its normal elasticity or snap-back resilience.

- Loss of the normal structural collagen support results in both deep and superficial wrinkles, which can be further aggravated by gravity, facial movement and sleeping positions.

- There is a moderate decrease in the number of blood vessels, which leads to impaired healing and slower removal of substances absorbed through skin, as well as loss of the normal pink complexion of youth.

- The sebaceous (oil) glands which produce a natural moisturizer become smaller and less numerous. This is good for those with oily, acne-prone skin, but eventually the skin becomes dry, which tends to excessively accentuate the most superficial wrinkles.

- Accumulation of the dead, dry skin layers on the surface and damage to skin fibers make skin texture more coarse and "bumpy."

- Loss of some pigment cells and increase in others causes uneven pigmentation.

- A reduction of immune cells is associated with fewer allergic reactions, but also a greater incidence of skin cancers.

- There is a gradual reduction in the number of hairs. Those that remain may be smaller, grow more slowly and often turn grey.

The list of skin changes goes on and on. The good news is that the majority of these changes are caused by sun exposure and can be readily prevented. Eventually, however, some of the changes described will occur even in those who protect their skin from the sun. But, the onset of such changes will occur later in life and will be much less severe.

Our Skin And The Sun

How The Sun Affects Our Skin

Sun damage causes our skin to age prematurely, and causes some skin cancers.

We have the French designer Coco Chanel to thank for the introduction of a tan as a 'healthy' accessory to smart dressing.

Fortunately, the trend now appears to be on its way out. Thanks to better public education and awareness of the dangers of too much sun, popularized and embodied by film stars such as Meryl Streep and Bette Midler, non-tanned skin is back in fashion.

Whether to tan or not is a matter of personal choice, not a prerequisite for looking healthy.

A *small* amount of low intensity sunlight is required by skin for the production of vitamin D. However, **there is no safe way of acquiring a tan, with or without sunscreen protection.**

Sunlight is made up of different colors of light. It is the ultraviolet (UV) light that is responsible for the majority of damage to the skin and skin immune system including immune cells called Langerhans cells. UV light concentration increases the closer the earth is to the sun. It is greatest at the equator, between 10 a.m. and 3 p.m., and in the height of summer. It is also greater where there is less atmosphere to absorb sun rays, such as at high altitude.

Reflective surfaces such as water, sand, snow and light-colored surfaces like metal or concrete will also increase the total dose of UV light by bouncing it back toward the body. UV light is itself composed of three types of rays.

Ultraviolet light C (UVC) is the most harmful. It is largely blocked by the ozone layer so that only minute amounts reach the earth's surface. Ultraviolet light B (UVB) is the one responsible for sunburn, tanning and skin cancers. It does not penetrate deeply into the skin but damages cells in the outer layers where skin cancers originate. Ultraviolet light A (UVA) has less potential to cause skin cancers but because it penetrates deeper into the skin, UVA can damage deeper tissues including circulating immune cells.

Unlike UVB, UVA light appears to remain strong and damaging

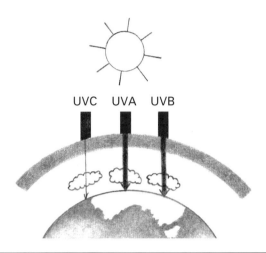

There are three types of ultraviolet light from the sun. UVC is the most harmful but is largely blocked by the ozone layer.

throughout the day and all year long. Researchers now believe that exposure to both UVA and UVB, may cause cancer of tissues other than the skin, due to effects on the immune system. Except in very dark individuals, an acquired tan does not offer significant protection against further exposure to UV light.

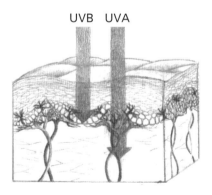

Both UVA and UVB light penetrate the skin. UVA goes deeper and can damage circulating immune cells. Both UVA and UVB can cause skin cancer.

Tanning Salons

The UV light delivered in tanning salons is mostly UVA light. Because of its deeper penetration into skin, UVA is now known to have damaging effects. It is not a safe way of acquiring a tan. There is no way of getting around it: **There is NO safe way of acquiring a tan by exposure to any UV light.**

Skin cancer is caused by UV light, not only by direct damage to individual skin cells, but also by impairment of the immune system. This allows cancerous cells to grow instead of being rejected and destroyed. There are three types of common skin cancers.

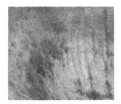 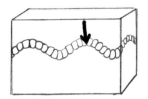

BASAL CELL CANCER

Basal cell cancer is a cancer of basal cells at the base of the epidermis. It starts as a small, red, itchy or scaly spot that does not heal. In the great majority of cases it will occur on the face and neck. This type almost never spreads to other organs and is therefore rarely fatal. However, it may grow to a large size requiring surgery. If treated early, it can be removed simply and easily by destroying with cautery (heat) and scraping, or freezing with liquid nitrogen spray. This is the most common of the skin cancers.

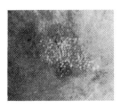 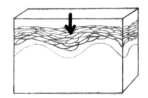

SQUAMOUS CELL CANCER

Squamous cell cancer is a cancer of cells in the outer epidermal layers. It also starts as a small scaly spot on any part of the body exposed to the sun and slowly grows with time. Unlike the basal cell cancer, it can spread to other organs and cause death. It can also be easily cured with early treatment in most cases.

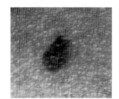 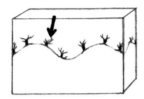

MELANOMA

Melanoma is a cancer of the pigment or tanning cells called melanocytes. It is the most dangerous of the skin cancers. It can spread even when small in size and result in unexpected and early death. Unlike the basal and squamous cell cancers which are almost always located in the sites most frequently exposed to the sun, melanoma can occur even in sites normally covered by clothing.

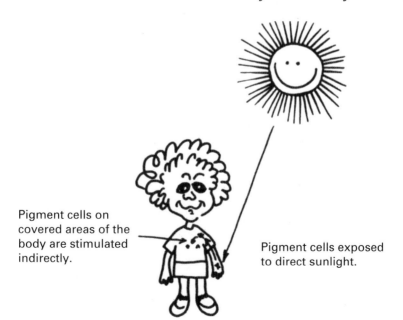

Pigment cells on covered areas of the body are stimulated indirectly.

Pigment cells exposed to direct sunlight.

A possible explanation for this is the indirect means by which melanocytes are stimulated by exposure to sunlight. Those pigment cells exposed to the sun in one part of the body such as the face and/or hands appear to produce a soluble substance that travels throughout the body and causes the rest of the pigment cells not directly exposed to the UV light to start producing more pigment. Thus, slightly abnormal pigment cells on areas of the body that are covered by clothing and thus protected from direct sunlight are still being stimulated to grow and multiply even in the absence of direct exposure to UV light.

Early complete removal, when the cancer is less than 0.75 mm thick, will usually result in a cure. If there is any suspicion about a pigmented spot being a melanoma, it should always be cut out and submitted to a lab for analysis to make sure that it is completely removed and to provide a true diagnosis. Any pigmented spot that changes color or size, itches or bleeds, should be checked by a physician.

Assymetry: one half of the mole is different to the other half.	Border irregularity: the edge or outline of the mole is uneven.	Color: mottled appearance, uneven shades of light and dark brown, black, red and even white.	Diameter: a mole or any growth on the skin larger than 6mm (¼ in.) in diameter should be a concern.

POSSIBLE WARNING SIGNS OF MELANOMA

HOW THE SUN AGES OUR SKIN

In addition to causing skin cancers, UV light accelerates aging of all skin layers. These aging effects increase in severity with greater exposure to the sun. In sun-damaged skin, wrinkles will appear earlier and will be deeper than would be expected with time alone.

To reduce the amount of UV light entering the skin, the body will increase the thickness of the superficial layers of the skin, especially the topmost, dead cell layer. This is a natural protective function and gives chronically sun-exposed skin a coarse, leathery texture and yellowish tone. Growth of pre-cancerous, scaly spots known as actinic keratoses, further adds to the uneven surface of the skin.

Frequent stimulation of the tanning cells will eventually lead to uneven or blotchy darker pigmentation (age spots), as well as white patches where tanning cells have died because of too much exposure to the sun.

Abnormal elastin fibers are produced and there is pronounced degradation of collagen, both of which cause deep wrinkles.

There is also a marked decrease in the number of healthy blood vessels and an increase in the number of tortuous enlarged vessels known as "broken capillaries." These capillaries can be seen through the top layers of skin as excessive redness.

Heat from sunlight can have a drying effect, which further compounds the damaging effects on the outer skin layers.

A quick way for you to assess the degree of sun damage is to compare your face, forearms, back of hands and neck to the skin on your buttocks (assuming you haven't been sun-bathing your buttocks!). If the skin on your arms is always darker, unevenly pigmented (both dark and white spots), has reddish background, or is dry and wrinkled in comparison to your buttocks, it is sun-damaged.

In sunny climates, such as California and Australia, severe sun damage (premature aging) can become visible as early as the teens and twenties. Hopefully, thanks to better education and healthier fashion trends, this degree of damage in young skin will not be seen as frequently in the future. Also, it is possible to remove some of the effects of sun damage such as broken capillaries and wrinkles and stimulate new collagen formation with specific laser techniques and other treatments (discussed in Chapters 7-9). However, prevention is always better than cure. We need to carefully consider all the harmful effects of the sun when deciding whether to sacrifice our health and appearance of our skin in the future for a tan today.

OTHER ENVIRONMENTAL STRESSES
Weather Conditions

Heat, cold, wind and low air humidity can all adversely affect our skin. All have a drying effect, especially on the outer layers.

To protect us against cold and wind, skin may become thicker.

Repeated heat and cold injury may eventually lead to the appearance of excess blood vessels (broken capillaries). Sudden changes from hot to cold conditions, and back again, as when we move between inside and outside in cold climates during winter, can be particularly damaging.

Sitting close to a heater or fire can also, after a prolonged period of time, cause purple mottling of the exposed skin. This is seen mostly in older people after many years of such exposure.

Older people are more susceptible to both heat and cold exposure. The effects are intensified by wind.

It is best to avoid extremes of temperature by wearing protective clothing and avoiding exposure to direct or high heat.

Excessive or prolonged exposure to cold temperatures can cause chilblains and frostbite. Chilblains are red, painful areas usually on the knuckles of hands or toes exposed to cold. Frostbite is the result of intense cold that freezes exposed skin and underlying tissues.

In air-conditioned or heated environments, humidifying the air may help prevent our skin from drying out. If you don't have a humidifier, a dish or bucket of water will suffice. Evaporation of water can be improved by dipping a piece of cloth or paper towel partly in the water and over the edge of the container. This also allows you to breathe more easily, especially if you are sensitive to dust or dryness.

Other ways to prevent dry skin are outlined in Chapter 5.

It is best to avoid excessive cleansing at any time. In winter, low humidity of both the cold outside air and heated indoor air can cause even normal or oily skin to become dry. Likewise, it is best to avoid prolonged or hot baths and showers. They strip the skin of the protective oily surface film. This needs to be replenished by applying a good body lotion, such as Amber Essence Face and Body Replenishing lotion, immediately after a shower or a bath.

The Sea

Salt water alone, without associated sun exposure, has little effect on the skin. The loss of moisture caused by salt water can be replenished by using appropriate moisturizers which are discussed in Chapter 5. It is more important to protect our skin from sunlight whenever we are near water because of the increased dose of UV light reflecting off the water and sand.

THE EFFECTS OF WEAR AND TEAR

Rubbing Skin

Continually removing and applying make-up, harsh abrasives and excessive use of exfoliative agents, can damage underlying collagen and elastin fibers. It is best to use only gentle scrubs, not to rub skin excessively, especially under the eyes where it is thin, and to apply moisturizers and cleansers by gently using fingertips or cotton ball applicators.

Sleeping Positions

How we sleep can also cause mechanical injury by repeatedly creasing certain areas of the face. For example, people who habitually lie on their stomach can develop vertical crease lines on their forehead. Those who favor sleeping on their side may develop deeper lines on the side of the face they usually sleep on.

Facial Expressions

There is some truth to the universally-used warning by mothers: "If you don't stop making that face, it will stay like that."

Deep wrinkles or folds develop in the skin overlying muscles used for making facial expressions. For example, frowning can produce deep furrows or *worry lines* on the forehead.

Lines caused by facial expressions are more difficult to correct with surgery or other methods. Because breaking the habit of a particular expression is very difficult, the lines are likely to return.

Your facial expressions automatically reflect your thoughts. Whether happy, sad or bored your face will usually show it unless like actors, you learn to control your expressions. You need not, however, go to such extremes.

The two worst culprits or wrinkle generators are frowning and squinting. Frowning can be reduced by becoming aware of the tension that usually causes it, and then consciously trying to relax the forehead muscles by gently massaging them with your fingers.

The most common cause of squinting is bright sunlight. A pair of sunglasses that filter UV light will help reduce squinting.

Another facial expression that causes lines is smiling. But please, don't stop smiling! Smiling will actually, physiologically make you feel happy.

Facial muscle exercises have been recommended by some as a helpful way of restoring waning muscle tone. Others, however, believe that any unnecessary facial muscle movements are harmful, because unlike in the rest of the body, facial muscles are attached directly to the overlying skin. This means that movement of the muscles will also move and stretch the skin. Excessive stretching may damage the underlying collagen and elastin fibers and worsen rather than improve wrinkles.

Such stretching of skin can be avoided, however, while still stimulating and toning muscles by means of externally applied electrical stimulation. This is discussed in detail in Chapter 4.

Gentle massage or facials are also helpful in relaxing the muscles and increasing circulation to the skin, provided they are not done too harshly or vigorously.

Frequent Weight Gain And Loss

Rapid gain and loss of 10 lbs. or more can damage the skin by stretching the superficial and deep connective tissues. This stretched tissue may return to its original size very slowly or on rare occasions, not at all.

The end result is that skin will sag and develop permanent stretch marks. Normal expression lines may become exaggerated, resulting in a droopy look earlier in life than would otherwise be expected.

Smoking And Alcohol

Both smoking and alcohol are damaging to skin. The effects of alcohol are less well defined than smoking. However, heavy alcohol consumption is often associated with smoking as well as poor diet — in particular vitamin B deficiency. Lack of vitamin B can result in dry, thin skin that is easily damaged and does not heal well. Both smoking and alcohol have a premature aging effect on the skin.

Heavy smokers will eventually develop a sallow, yellowish complexion and more wrinkles than would normally be expected for their age. These effects are caused by nicotine which has a retarding effect on cell growth in the skin and reduces blood supply. Thus, a smoker's skin will heal more slowly and not as well as, that of a non-smoker. Some wrinkles, for example, the *smoker's lines* around the lips, are also caused partly by the repeated facial expressions associated with smoking. If smoking is discontinued, some of these effects may partially reverse in time.

Smoking is also an environmental hazard for those who don't smoke but who live with heavy smokers, or work in cigarette smoke-filled environments. Passive smoking can affect skin in the same way it affects smokers.

It is a popular misconception that heavy alcohol intake is associated with the appearance of broken capillaries on the nose and cheeks. This is merely a coincidental finding. People are more likely to develop a *red nose* or broken capillaries because of familial predisposition or sun damage, not because of alcohol. Alcohol has a dilating effect on superficial blood vessels and can therefore make existing capillaries appear more prominent. It does not, however, cause them.

Sun damage can cause the appearance of broken capillaries by damaging collagen and elastin fibers. This allows the underlying blood vessels to grow unimpeded, too close to the surface of the skin where the red blood circulating through the excess vessels makes them easily visible. These excess blood vessels are not needed for the normal function of skin and can be removed with medical treatments (see Chapter 9).

Nutrition

What we eat also affects our skin but in more subtle ways. Foods high in fat content do not cause acne but may make it worse. Similarly, hot spicy foods may make broken capillaries temporarily appear more prominent by dilating them with increased blood flow.

All tissues, including the skin, will suffer from poor nutrition. In the skin, lack of vitamin C can result in easy bruising and poor healing and vitamin B deficiency can cause dry, thin skin. Such severe vitamin deficiencies are unusual in most prosperous communities, because of supplements in bread, milk and other foods.

Eating balanced meals is essential for keeping ourselves nutritionally healthy.

THE FREE RADICAL THEORY OF AGING

Scientists believe that the genetically-set maximum life span is about 120 years and that it is free radicals which prevent us from living this long. Denham Harman was the first to postulate the free radical theory of aging more than thirty years ago. As with most new discoveries based on theory, not much attention was paid to it. In 1969, two biochemists proved beyond doubt that free radicals are present throughout our body and since then, free radicals have been extensively researched.

All matter is made of particles called molecules, which in turn are composed of even smaller parts called atoms. An atom consists of: a central nucleus and orbiting electrons. Normally electrons are found in pairs. Loss of an electron, which happens everyday in our bodies dur-

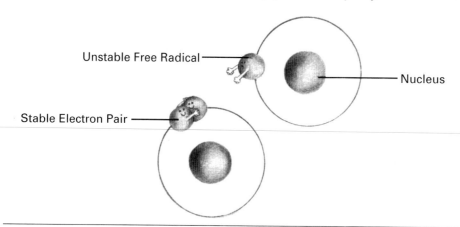

Unstable Free Radical

Nucleus

Stable Electron Pair

Molecules are made up of a nucleus and orbiting electrons which usually form pairs. An unstable molecule has unpaired electrons called free radicals which can disrupt tissue by trying to steal an electron from a stable molecule.

ing metabolism, (the tissue utilization of food and oxygen) and the body's detoxification of a vast variety of chemicals, results in molecules becoming unstable.

It is then called a free radical. It disrupts tissue, including the genetic content of cells, by stealing an electron from the nearest molecule, which in turn steals an electron from its neighbor. This initiates the domino effect or chain reaction. If it were not kept under control by substances called antioxidants, it would cause major damage in our bodies. Fortunately, most of the damage is not lethal. However, it is cumulative and can in time lead to many of the health-related changes and problems we associate with age, including cancer, heart and lung disease, cataracts, Parkinson's and even Alzheimer's disease.

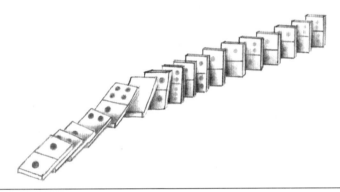

Free radicals cause a domino effect on tissue by "stealing" electrons from stable molecules and thus, in turn, destabilizing them.

It is impossible to prevent free radicals from forming since they are by-products of our normal bodily functions. However, it is possible to reduce their formation by being aware that burnt (charred) meat or toast, rancid butter or oils, deep fried foods, smoking, alcohol, sun exposure, especially sunburn, and a whole range of medications as well as stress stimulate free radical formation.

Limiting the total amount of fats eaten is a very important step in combating free radicals. This is because fats are more susceptible to free radical formation than either protein or carbohydrates, both before and after they are eaten.

For years, we have been told that unsaturated fats are better than saturated fats: by lowering cholesterol, they prevent heart disease. They do, but they also appear to be more susceptible to free radical formation by reacting with oxygen, especially during cooking. The solution is to cut total fat intake to 15% of the total calories and no more than 30%. Do not fry foods and especially avoid deep frying. If you absolutely have to fry, use as little oil as possible for as short a time as possible.

The result of the action of oxygen in the atmosphere on foods exposed to it, is the formation of free radicals. A visible example of this is the browning of apples or potatoes cut and left exposed to the air. Some foods oxidize more than others. Unsaturated fats appear to be the most susceptible but all foods will eventually oxidize. This can be prevented by eating or cooking fruits and vegetables as soon as they are cut, covering them in plastic food wrap or submerging them in cold water in an airtight container. All food, fresh and canned, should be similarly protected from the air. Do not eat any food that has become rancid or otherwise spoiled.

It is also possible to prevent, or at least reduce, the damaging effects of free radicals by eating foods that contain antioxidants. Antioxidants include vitamins A, C and E, selenium and zinc, among others.

Vitamin A (beta-carotene) is found naturally in many fruits and vegetables, especially those which are orange or red in color, such as carrots, sweet potatoes, apricots and mangos. Too much vitamin A can be toxic. Dry skin, irritability, headache, loss of hair and, in very high doses, liver problems are side effects from toxic dosage.

Vitamin C (ascorbic acid) is the water-soluble equivalent of vitamin E. Vitamin C neutralizes free radicals inside the watery content of cells. It has been postulated that the two compounds that form as a result of vitamin C combining with free radicals may have their own anti-cancer properties.

Vitamin C is found in most fresh fruits and vegetables. However, high enough doses may not be obtained from just eating these foods to combat free radicals, when under additional stress such as physical injury, surgery, burns, infection and pregnancy.

Humans, unlike most mammals, are not able to manufacture vitamin C in response to stress. Dogs, for example, make as much as 4,000 mg per hour when exposed to stress. Extra vitamin C, therefore, needs to be ingested under stressful conditions. Doctors vary in their recommendations as to optimal doses. Some recommend 500 mg, some 2,000 mg or more daily. Very high doses of vitamin C have been found to result in kidney stones if water intake is not adequate.

It is best to check with your doctor or nutritionist before embarking on a vitamin supplement program, as each of us has individual requirements that may change over time. These may be more accurately gauged by blood biochemistry analysis.

Vitamin E is fat-soluble. It is found naturally in nuts, seeds, seed oils, wheat germ and lobster. Vitamin E sits between the fatty layers that compose cell membranes (or walls), where it is ideally situated to protect cells from free radicals, which threaten to damage the cells from inside and outside.

Vitamin E can actually prolong the life of a cell. This is especially important in maintaining good immune functions. Do not assume, however, that the more you take, the healthier you will be. Too much vitamin E can be harmful. It can prolong bleeding time and should be discontinued two weeks before surgery. Since the foods containing vitamin E also have a fairly high fat content, it may be advisable to eat some and supplement these with extra Vitamin E in capsule form. The recommended dose is 200 international units (I.U.), and no more than 600 I.U. daily.

Selenium indirectly eliminates free radicals called peroxides by aiding in the production of an enzyme which converts these free radicals into water. Other than its general anti-radical function, selenium appears to protect against heart disease. Selenium is found in whole grains, bread, cereals, seafood and in vegetables such as cabbage, broccoli, celery, onions and mushrooms. The content of selenium in these vegetables will vary depending on where they were grown. It may be wise to take extra selenium but not more than 100-200 micrograms daily. Higher doses can cause nausea, diarrhea, and even nerve damage.

Zinc works both indirectly by being part of an enzyme and directly, to protect cells from free radicals. Zinc can be obtained from a variety of foods including beef, liver, nuts and cheeses. However, since these foods also have a fairly high fat content, which is not desirable, supplements of only 15-30 mg per day may be advisable. Doses of 15 mg a day enhance immune function by, among others, restoring production of thymic hormones that regulate the immune system and increasing the activity of natural killer cells. Too much can cause nausea, vomiting and general gastro-intestinal irritation.

Scientists are talking about developing synthetic enzymes which will be able to prevent the damage caused by free radicals and repair the genetic damage that already occurred. In practical terms, this would mean repairing cells whose genes have become damaged; in other words, finding the cure for cancer.

THE GROWTH HORMONE THEORY OF AGING

The human growth hormone has recently gained attention as having possible anti-aging potential. The hormone is normally manufactured by part of our brain, a small gland called the pituitary. It is especially important in childhood, determining how fast and how much we grow. Once growth is completed, the hormone appears to direct its attention to regulating the amount of fat and muscle. Lower levels of the hormone occur as we grow older, resulting in middle-age spread, increased fat and less muscle. This eventually leads to loss of strength as seen in the elderly.

A report in the *New England Journal Of Medicine* several years ago, suggested that synthetic human growth hormone was responsible for making volunteers – aged 61 to 81 years – physiologically as much as ten years younger after six months of treatment.

The growth hormone is currently used to treat children who lack the hormone and would otherwise remain very short in stature. It has not been approved for use as anti-aging medication. There are many questions yet to be answered including possible side-effects, whether it works in women as well as men, the optimal age at which to start taking the hormone and whether it can help people whose growth hormone levels are normal.

A word of caution: there is an illegal source of growth hormone of doubtful quality and potentially serious side-effects similar to those caused by steroids.

The Role Of Our Thoughts In Aging

Since our thoughts affect every aspect of our life, it is foreseeable that our thinking by means of releasing certain chemical substances or preventing the release of others, could slow down or even reverse the aging process. There is much yet to be learned about the potential of the human mind!

Reach Out

The Institute for the Advancement of Health recently found that people who performed volunteer work regularly for at least two hours, once a week, were ten times more likely to be in good health compared to those who didn't. Becoming involved in helping others was also associated with a sense of well-being and fewer stress-related problems.

CHAPTER

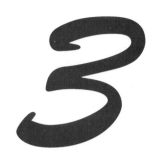

Nutrition And Dieting

People of America, the greatest threat to the survival of you and your children is not some terrible nuclear weapon. It is what you are going to eat from your dinner plate tonight.

David Reuben

Today we are eating healthier than our parents did. Unfortunately, a preoccupation with weight and dieting has come hand-in-hand with the more positive change. The social pressure to be thin is the reason why so many women with perfectly normal bodies see themselves as being too fat and start dieting.

Did you know that excessive depression, anxiety and even sleep disturbances may result from excessive dieting. In fact, obsession with weight and chronic dieting have been identified as the most common forms of emotional disorders in women today.

Think about how many times we have, in fact, gone hungry simply for the sake of appearance, depriving our body of its nourishment. Humans are unique in the animal kingdom. No other animal starves itself to be thin.

I agree with Dr. Rita Freedman, whose central theme in her book *Bodylove* is that "you shouldn't have to suffer or torment your body in order to feel better about your looks and yourself."

Body structure is largely determined by genetic factors, not simply by exercising self-control and working at it. To achieve the super slim figures of the 20-year-old models is not realistic. It would, for most people, require the loss of muscle as well as fat. While this is possible, at least temporarily, it requires an almost super-human effort, and is often doomed to failure from the beginning.

Our body is a most marvelous conception whose built-in survival mechanism counterbalances weight reduction, which is too fast or excessive, by lowering the metabolic rate. That is, reducing the expenditure of energy and stimulating cravings for high energy foods.

Eventually, when this built-in, automatic, self-preservation mechanism overrides the restraint and food deprivation to which we subjected ourselves, the combination of more efficient utilization and increased consumption of the very foods we have been trying to avoid, will result in weight gain beyond that present at the start.

Anorexia is a disorder in which this survival mechanism fails to halt and reverse the effects of starvation. Without medical intervention, this can lead to weight loss so extreme, it can result in death. Anorexia is just one of the many types of eating disorders prevalent today.

In an attempt to gain pseudo self-esteem, we forget or don't realize that:

> *Fat is not a measure of self-worth and neither is*
> *being thin an antidote to feeling fat!*
>
> **Rita Freedman**

True self-worth is based on making rational decisions that best ensure our survival and enhance our well being.

It is also based on our ability to **trust** ourselves to consistently make such positive, realistic choices.

Excessive, unrealistic dieting is the opposite of these healthy choices. It only serves to deplete self-worth.

Unfortunately, the word "diet" has become associated with the thousands of different but unrealistic attempts at weight reduction by means of distorted eating patterns.

The "all protein diet," "all fruit" or just plain starvation diet, have all been tried and in the long run failed. If "dieting" means depriving the body of necessary nutrients, it is best not to "diet" at all.

This is exactly the advice of Dr. Nancy Bonus who over the last twenty years has developed a non-diet, permanent weight loss program called *The Bonus Plan — Food Without Fear*. It is based on building healthy self-esteem, not destroying it, by learning to make rational, healthy but tasty choices. The only condition of the *Bonus Plan* is that you eat whatever you want *and* enjoy it. It really works. My own experience with dieting confirms this approach. I lost 30 pounds **only after I stopped dieting** and started eating whatever I wanted whenever I wanted. Unencumbered by punishment resulting from too much restraint, it was amazing how quickly my rational decision-making took over and returned eating habits to healthy *and* tasty *choices.*

The word "diet" comes from the Greek work diaita, which means "a way of life." This is a good concept to follow.

The best food plan is considerate and gentle on our stomach, and nutritious for our body. We need to eat only food that is healthy and supplies us with enough nutrients and calories to maintain optimum health. Any excess calories we consume will be stored as fat, and consuming any less than required is likely to make us feel hungry and reduce our energy and frustration level.

Not all calories, however, are of equal value. Calories derived from fruit will be utilized differently and are more valuable than those derived from refined carbohydrates such as white flour and sugar. The lack of fiber and nutrients makes the latter foods "empty" calories.

If we want to have a slimmer figure, we first need to decide what is a reasonable amount to lose, then try to lose it slowly. No more than 1-2 lbs. a week, incorporating new habits which are likely to keep the fat off on a more permanent basis. For example, increasing our expenditure of calories by exercising in addition to reducing the number of calories eaten.

Remember, excessive reduction in calories eaten may result in loss of muscle in addition to fat. This is not the goal of a healthy diet. The aim is to reduce the stored fat and therefore inches off the storage areas, not total body weight. Muscle weighs more than fat and a large percentage (70-90 percent) of the body tissues contain water. Loss of muscle and dehydration will result in loss of total weight but not necessarily loss of the excess fatty deposits.

In general, 3,500 calories are equivalent to about one pound of fat. Thus, reducing our intake by 250 calories a day will allow us to lose about half a pound a week.

This may not sound like very much. **Dieters** are notoriously impatient. Think of it this way, if you had started a year ago, you could now weigh 26 pounds less. Assuming, of course, that you had this much excess fat to lose.

It is easier to go on short-term fad diets than to alter thinking consistently enough to change habits of behavior, to make daily healthy choices.

When we treat our body with respect, it rewards us with good health, vitality and a less stressful and more enjoyable life. However, if we put our body on a starvation diet, it will punish us with difficult to control cravings for *forbidden, fattening* food, excessive tiredness, bad moods and depression.

The choice seems clear — but where do we begin?

How about with attitude. If we are not already eating well, we first need to look at the reasons why not.

Do we eat out of boredom, loneliness, frustration? Some foods do affect our moods.

For example, tryptophan, a naturally occurring amino acid is converted to serotonin in the brain.

Serotonin is one of the neurotransmitters or brain juices discussed in Chapter 1 which can affect our mood. It promotes relaxation and makes us feel more relaxed to the point of feeling sleepy. A high carbohydrate and low protein meal enhances the production of serotonin.

Thus, certain food cravings can be stimulated by physiological and emotional factors.

To avoid or reduce such cravings, it is important to eat some carbohydrates throughout the day. However, remember a high carbohydrate meal will make us relaxed and sleepy.

When we want to maintain a sharp, clear focus, we need to eat more protein and less carbohydrate.

Once we have ascertained reasons why we may be eating inappropriately, determine to correct and change them.

Invariably, this is going to involve what and how we think.

Following are some self-talk suggestions which, if repeated daily, will gradually help to change our outlook and attitude about our weight and appearance:

> *I choose to eat food that ensures my perfect health and my ideal weight.*

> *I eat just enough to keep my ideal weight and leave excess food on my plate in front of me.*

> *I enjoy eating good tasting, healthy foods.*

> *I love the way I look and feel.*

Whatever other self-talk statements you make, always put them in the present — not the future. Also, make the statements positive rather than negative. For example, it is better to say "I eat only healthy food," rather than say "I do not eat any food that is not good for me."

PRINCIPLES OF A HEALTHY DIET

Eating Habits

- We need to eat for energy and health. To supply our body with all the nutrients it needs and cut down on the extras it doesn't need.

- It is best to eat slowly and chew our food well. It takes about twenty minutes from the time food reaches our stomach to feel satisfied. We will continue to feel hungry and overeat if we eat a meal in ten minutes, even if we have eaten too much. Hot soups may curb our appetite. Since they are hot, they have to be eaten slowly.

- It is better to eat small meals more frequently: three small meals a day, with two or three snacks in between, rather than one or two large meals. It is preferable to eat the last meal of the day before 6 p.m., if possible.

- It is also preferable to eat only at the kitchen or dining room table.

It is especially important to avoid snacking in front of the television.

- It is advisable to eat before going grocery shopping. This prevents our hunger from doing the shopping for us.

In General Do Eat

- Fresh fruit and vegetables daily.

- Fish twice a week.

- Red meat, not more than one-to-two times a week or not at all.

- White meat such as chicken or turkey two-to-three times a week or less.

- Non-fat, or low-fat, dairy products.

- High-fiber foods, at least one ounce (35 grams) of fiber a day, but no more than two ounces (60 grams).

- Drink plenty of water every day (6 glasses, more when exercising).

It is important that we eat what we like. The idea of healthy food habits is to provide us with nourishment and satisfaction. If we don't like a particular fruit or vegetable or food-type, we don't have to eat it, even if it is supposed to be good for us.

Do Not Eat

- Saturated fats, such as animal fats in meat, milk and butter. These fats increase our blood cholesterol level, and weight-for-weight, contain twice as many calories as protein or carbohydrate.

- Refined carbohydrates, such as products made of white flour, sugar and alcohol. These are loaded with *empty* calories, which are devoid of most natural nutrients.

Cooking Hints

- Plan meals around whole grains, vegetables and fruits. Think of meat as a garnish or side dish.

- Purchase only lean meat and trim off all visible fat before cooking, as fat is less easily visible after cooking.

- Remove skin from poultry, as most of the fat is in the skin. This can be easily done after cooking. The skin keeps the meat moist without apparently adding calories.

- Reduce added fats in favorite recipes by substituting light sour cream or yogurt for butter and cream, and mustard for mayonnaise.

- Use non-stick cooking spray or non-stick cookware instead of oil and butter.

- Grill, roast or poach meats but avoid charring them as this may add free radicals to your diet.

- Grill or roast red meats instead of frying them since no additional oil or butter is required and excess fat from the meat will drip away during cooking.

- Steam vegetables.

Special Food Considerations

Fats

Not only has fat twice as many calories as protein or carbohydrate, but it is also less efficiently utilized. Only 3-5 percent of fat calories are burnt by our body after these substances are eaten, compared to 20-25 percent of the calories in carbohydrates. The number of calories that the body continues to burn at rest after a carbohydrate meal is also slightly higher than that after a fatty meal.

Fats are difficult to give up because they add flavor. It is fat that carries and releases the flavor of spices in food. It is a matter of re-educating our palate to limit fat to no more than 15-30 percent of our caloric intake. This means that every 100 calories eaten contain no more than 0.1 ounce (3 grams) of fat.

Fats can be saturated, such as fat found in meat, butter, eggs and full-fat dairy products. Polyunsaturated, as found in vegetable oils or monounsaturated as in oils from seeds, nuts vegetables and some fish.

Saturated fats are required for the body to function normally. However, our bodies are able to manufacture almost all of the saturated fats they need. Any saturated fats obtained in our diet are not required and cause trouble.

Excess saturated fats cause high cholesterol which, with the help of free radicals, lead to problems like clogging of arteries and heart disease. Blood cholesterol levels of 200 mg or more are too high and are associated with a significantly greater risk of heart disease, including heart attack.

High levels of other fats called triglycerides and low density lipoproteins (LDL — fat partially mixed with protein) are also harmful. However, not all fats are bad. Polyunsaturated and monounsaturated fats are good. By displacing saturated fats, they in fact neutralize their negative effects. They can also decrease blood pressure and improve kidney function.

A low fat diet alone will lower cholesterol but **it can also lower good fats**, high density lipoproteins (HDL), **and raise levels of triglycerides.**

A diet containing monounsaturated fats (such as found in peanut and olive oils) can lower cholesterol without lowering the good HDLs or raising triglycerides. Another one of these good fats is found in fish, particularly cold water fish. It is called Omega-3. It has the unique ability to actually lower the harmful triglyceride blood levels.

A twenty-year study in Holland demonstrated that men who ate at least 1 ounce (30 grams) of fish per day, had half the incidence of heart disease compared to men who did not eat any fish. For those who dislike fish, Omega-3 can be obtained in the form of capsules. It is also found in some plant oils in the form of linoleic acid.

Ideally, about one-third of the fat we eat can be saturated, one-third polyunsaturated and the remainder monounsaturated.

Protein

Protein should constitute about 15% of our diet unless we are under conditions of stress, such as surgery or other injury including skin ulceration when more than this may be required. Any increase in protein intake, however, should be moderate, especially in older people, as the kidneys may not be able to handle large amounts of protein.

Protein appears to enhance calcium absorption which is needed for normal bone formation and maintenance. However, if protein exceeds 20% of the diet, calcium may actually be lost in the urine.

In general, it is best to obtain protein from plants, nuts, fish and white, rather than red meat. However, do not rely too heavily on just vegetables in your diet. This can lead to loss of estrogen in bowel movements which can contribute towards bone weakness called osteoporosis.

Carbohydrate And Fiber

The best way to obtain carbohydrates is from fruits, vegetables and whole grains. In addition to containing fewer calories and more nutrition than sugar alone (high in carbohydrate), they also contain fiber.

Fiber helps to curb appetite by taking longer to chew so that our stomach has time to register as full. Once in the stomach, fiber attracts water and expands, filling the stomach and further reducing hunger.

Fiber also slows down the absorption of sugar and consequently slows down the rise in insulin which is released in response to sugar in blood. Insulin can trigger the feeling of hunger.

Fiber can also actually reduce the calories eaten by about 5%, by removing some fats before they have had a chance to be absorbed. This could amount to as much as 100 calories per day. As you can see, fiber is not only healthy, but can be of great help when trying to lose excess body fat.

As with everything that is good for you, don't overdo it. Too much fiber (more than 30-60 grams a day) can bind calcium, making it unavailable for absorption, which can lead to osteoporosis.

Calcium

Calcium is required for optimal health of bones, teeth, nerve and muscle cells. It also helps blood to clot normally, for example, after a cut to the skin. Osteoporosis (caused by lack of calcium) is a lifestyle problem which can lead to serious consequences, including multiple bone fractures. Although not directly related to the health of skin, this condition is very much related to aging and nutrition.

If the only dairy product you take is milk in your coffee, you are likely to require an additional source of calcium. But, caffeine, tobacco, red meat, too much protein or fiber, and soft drinks, if taken at the same time as calcium (as supplements or dairy products), can inhibit its absorption from the intestine.

Furthermore, milk products eaten together with meat (for example, cream sauces) will result not only in calcium from the milk not being absorbed, but also the iron in meat (needed for red blood cell formation) not being available in a form that is easily absorbed.

The optimal intake of calcium is 1000-1500 mg a day; however, higher doses of 2000 mg a day appear to have anti-colon cancer properties by reducing intestinal cell activity. One 8 fl ounce (250 ml) glass of skim milk contains 300 mg.

See your doctor or nutritionist if you have any doubts about your calcium intake. If you are concerned about the health of your bones, you can have bone density studies to diagnose osteoporosis.

Water

> *A camel can lose 8 percent of its body weight in fluid before it is physically in danger. A donkey can tolerate 5 percent loss of its body weight before it is at risk. Human beings, however, can tolerate only 3 percent loss of body weight before risking collapse, kidney damage, and other impairments.*
>
> Betty Hennessy

Water Requirements During Exercise

A person who weighs 150 lbs. could lose 3 percent of body water after just an hour and a half of strenuous activity, such as running.

If this is not replaced at 20 minute intervals by taking eight to twelve sips of water, rehydration will not occur during continued strenuous activity, even if all the water is replaced in the second hour.

It is therefore very important to replace water lost by sweating at regular, short intervals, *while* it is being lost, not just after.

Daily Water Requirements

Daily water losses without exercise include:

- Two cups through lungs

- Two cups through sweating

- Six cups through intestines and kidneys

- Total: Ten Cups

Daily water intake includes, approximately:

- 3½ cups in our food

- ½ cup as by-product of metabolism

- Total: Four Cups

We therefore need to drink about six cups a day when we do not exercise.

Exercise significantly increases our water requirement. Dr. Hennessy suggests that during strenuous activity, we should develop the habit of drinking eight to twelve swallows of water every twenty minutes or so.

What We Drink

Fluids we drink stay in the stomach until the stomach adds enough salts to the fluid so that it is the same consistency as the fluids in the intestines or if the fluid is already salty or sweet, adds water to dilute it.

It is therefore important not to drink fluids that are too sweet or salty, especially during exercise, as this may further dehydrate our body.

A concentration of salts or sugar of about five to eight percent appears to be ideal.

Water Terminology*

Purified Water

Water is purified when it contains less than ten parts per million (ppm) of total dissolved solids (tds) or minerals.

Most tap water contains about 400-600 ppm of tds. This varies depending on the geographical area.

The term "purified" has **nothing** to do with cleanliness or bacterial count of the water. Few consumers realize this and mistake purified water for something which is completely clean and microbially safe. Hence, costly bottled "designer" water may be purified, but may have plenty of bacteria in it, if it is packed in a plastic bottle, since all plastic breathes.

Some purified bottled waters have very high bacterial counts, which is why after a few months it is necessary to discard the water and replace it because eventually the bacterial load is so great that algae begins to form. Bacteria need light and air to multiply and all plastic bottles have both. This is not to say that drinking bottled water is necessarily harmful; nearly all foods and beverages contain some bacteria. It is dangerous, though, if pathogenic bacteria are present. Excessive levels of even non-pathogenic bacteria, found in nearly all bottled water, indicate that the water must be discarded after several months.

"Spring Water" can start out pure but if the source of the water is not a spring, it can still benefit from being purified. Two very common ways are Reverse Osmosis (RO) or Deionization (DI). Deionization is generally more thorough and is the way Aqua Blox® water is purified. Its tds count is well below 10 ppm; usually between 1-3 ppm tds. It is carbon filtered multiple times. This filtration removes all chlorine from the water.

Distilled Water

The distillation process will render any grade of water purified, and at the time of distillation, sterile. However, after distillation, the water is usually packed into non-sterile jugs, bottles, or other containers which inherently contain some bacteria and possibly other micro-organisms.

* Courtesy of AQUA Blox®

This means the water is no longer sterile, but it will be purified unless the vessel into which it is placed contains minerals or other residual matter.

The distillation process can use water from any source, no matter how contaminated, and yields purified and sterile water. Water is heated to 212 degrees Fahrenheit (boiling) and the resultant vapor is channeled into a receiving tank. It is the vapor that becomes the distilled water. All minerals, solids and non-viable micro-organisms are left behind in the beginning vessel.

Again, unless the container into which the distilled water is placed is sterile, the distilled water will not remain sterile. Plastic bottles cannot keep oxygen out and therefore cannot be sterile.

Aqua Blox® water is both purified and sterile and has a five-year shelf life. The water is heated to destroy all micro-organisms and is put into a sterile environment (its package) impervious to air or light. This prevents the water from becoming contaminated. It is ideal to keep in the home or at work, in case of emergencies, especially in earthquake-prone California.

Mineral Water

Mineral water must contain at least 50 ppm minerals (tds) which means it is definitely not purified; it may or may not be sterile but sterile mineral waters are uncommon.

Mineral water has benefits and many mineral water companies purposely add certain minerals in specific quantities to add flavor. Magnesium and calcium add a pleasant taste, described by water experts as "crisp." Manufacturers must disclose which minerals are found in their water and their relative percentages.

Treated Water

Treated water is made by adding chemicals to water so that it can be stored for extended periods. The chemicals essentially preserve the water by inhibiting bacterial growth. There are problems with treated water, not the least of which is unsavory taste. Studies suggest that children are unlikely to drink water with an off-taste even under emergency conditions, and can become dehydrated as a result of having only treated water on hand in an emergency.

Sterile Water

Sterile water does not contain viable organisms. Water sterility is usually attained through pasteurization, which means heating the water for a time period and temperature sufficient to kill all micro-organisms. Once organisms are dead they are harmless and are not part of the bacterial count on the lab report. This is referred to as "commercial" sterility. For example, Aqua Blox® is commercially sterile.

The other form of food/drug sterility is "pharmaceutical." The applications for pharmaceutical sterility in the medical industry for injectable drugs require a sterile material free of any organic matter. Pharmaceutical sterility is extremely costly and unnecessary for food or consumable water products.

Pharmaceutical sterility must also rely on micron filtration to remove microscopic organisms after their viability has been destroyed by heat.

Themarox™

Since about 1960, scientists have known that a rock called vermiculite has water-cleansing properties. Composed of at least 22 natural minerals which are not toxic to man, vermiculite is able to absorb organic and any attached toxic contaminants from water.

Asao Shimanishi in Japan is the scientist who developed a patented process of converting the mineral extract from vermiculite into a liquid form.

In polluted water, organic substances which adhere to water molecules are the contaminants, not the water molecules themselves. These organic substances which exist on water molecules are soluble. If these molecules were to become insoluble, the organic substances and whatever pollutants are attached to them, could be separated and removed, leaving clean water.

When a small amount of Themarox™ is added to polluted water, it acts as a catalyst to decompose organic substances into insoluble matter or flock which can be easily removed.

This has been used in Japan to clean fisheries, aquariums, sewage tanks and treatment plants, pools, public baths or any contaminated water and to improve quality of water used in agriculture. Themarox™ is being introduced to United States for the same purposes.

Themarox™ certainly seems to be nature's answer to the water pollution for which we are responsible and will warm the hearts of all concerned for our environment.

CHAPTER

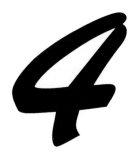

How To Deal With Stress

Just think what kind of world it would be if we all realized that we could be powerful in everything we do without being tense and rigid.

George Leonard

Our lives have become so complex that unless we make a determined effort to master our reactions to our environment, it will master us instead. The result is a feeling of stress, that is mental, emotional, or physical tension, strain or distress. Stress is a consequence of thinking and feeling disempowerment.

Unfortunately, we are often unaware of the virtually constant feeling of pressure generated by the thoughts and feelings of not being able to adequately control the many minor and often unavoidable frustrations we encounter every day.

The very technology which was created to make life easier for us, often seems to intensify these daily stresses by presenting us with so many different situations we need to handle in quick succession, that unless our mind is very agile as well as powerful and our thinking based on solid principles, we may succumb to the pressure of external influences.

Just as an athlete needs physical strength, so we need emotional, mental and spiritual muscle to master our environment and thus avoid stress. Our thinking needs to:

> *Be like the promontory against which the waves continually break, but which stands firm and tames the fury of the water around it.*
>
> **Aurelius**

The only way our thinking can be this strong and unshakable is when it is based on and guided by principles of integrity which in most religions and societies are defined by the ten commandments.

The strength of integrity and these value-based principles or code of correct conduct provide us with a system we can always depend on and which when followed always ensures consistent right thoughts and actions.

Without such a system, good thoughts and deeds would be random acts resulting from the arbitrary discretion of each individual.

To imagine the result, first imagine what our life would be like if there were no legal system or no police to keep law and order and we all depended on each other's goodwill.

People often complain about "the system." Based on the ten commandments, it is not the system that is at fault, but people's lack of adherence to right conduct that causes problems.

It goes without saying that what follows in the rest of this chapter first and foremost requires living up to standards set by the positive, ethical and moral value system of our society.

Without this baseline, attempting to change our thinking from negative to positive is like filling up a bottomless bucket with water.

They are aids which can help to center us in an ever more demanding world but they cannot provide us *with* the center. This center is the moral and spiritual fibre of our *character.*

Apart from feeling unpleasant, stress has deleterious effects on our body. The feeling of pressure sets off an automatic chain reaction in our body.

Our body responds to stress by releasing adrenalin, our blood pressure rises, muscles become tense and the nervous system is stimulated to make us feel more alert but also more anxious.

Prolonged stress adversely affects the immune system, which may reduce the body's ability to fight infections as well as possibly cancerous changes. Stress can also lead to insomnia, high blood pressure and even contribute to heart disease. It shows on the face with pronounced expression lines.

Everyone is vulnerable to stress. While it is impossible to avoid potentially stressful situations altogether, it is possible to alter the way we perceive and respond to them.

The first thing to do is to become aware of the sources of stress in our life. Make a list of the things that you find stressful. Then deal with the underlying causes.

We can reduce stress encountered during our daily activities by using our conscious mind to filter out the vast number of minor aggravations and focusing on the task at hand.

Planning time efficiently is also a way of reducing stress. As are setting priorities and saying "no" to things we cannot comfortably accomplish in the time we have allotted. The following are some of the strategies available to reduce or eliminate stress.

THE POWER OF 'NO'

How much less stress would we experience in life if we said "**NO**" to:

- Demands for material possessions.

- People who expect more from us than they are willing to give us or people who demand a free ride.

- People demanding approval and attention.

- People unloading their troubles onto us.

- People who say flattering things to our face to obtain a favor and stab us in the back with gossip.

- Nervous inability to make a commitment.

- Idle waste of time.

When you first learn to say "**NO**," you can expect to experience a little more stress initially:

> *Since those who request something from you hope for a **yes**, they may react in a negative manner to your **NO**. But any anger or sarcasm on their part is their problem. You must not let them make you feel that you have done something wrong. The opposite is true. You have done something right.*

> *Don't let anyone cause you to become doubtful or irritable. The denied person will sense this as the weakness that it is, and weakness is an invitation for the schemer to come and get it. You are the it. Once having said **NO**, you need only remain in the power and the wisdom of this spiritual atmosphere. This keeps you firm but polite, uncompromising and innocent.*

> *As you start to say **NO** to people, you see more clearly the nature of your true interests. And the more clearly you see what is truly best for you, the stronger becomes your **NO**.*
>
> Vernon Howard

TIME OUT

To take time out for ourselves is treating ourselves with respect and consideration. Giving ourselves some time off to enjoy our life, helps us accomplish our goals more effectively.

> *Often times in denying yourself pleasure you do but store the desire in the recesses of your being.*

> *Who knows but that which seems omitted today, waits for tomorrow?*

> *Even your body knows its heritage and its right-*

ful need and will not be deceived.

And your body is the harp of your soul,

And it is yours to bring forth sweet music from it or confused sounds.

Kahlil Gibran

MASSAGE AND FACIALS

Pamper yourself, for example, with a massage, a facial, or a relaxing bath (but not too hot or too long as this can result in the skin becoming too dry). Massage will help to relax tense muscles and has the additional benefits of increasing circulation to the skin and helping lymph fluid to drain. This aids the removal of waste substances from the skin.

In addition to the physiological benefits, touching also serves a psychological need of human contact, often healing, and is an antidote to the dehumanizing aspects of an increasingly technological society.

RELAXATION

We tend to think of relaxation as being a passive non-activity until we try to relax. We then find that it may take some effort to do so. The amount of effort depends on the degree of stress we feel at the time.

The full expression of empowerment requires thinking with calm command. That is, a state of mind that is relaxed.

In his book *The Relaxation Response,* Dr. Herbert Benson suggests the following method, which when practiced often enough will help us develop the habit of being able to relax at will.

1. Sit quietly in a comfortable position.

2. Close your eyes.

3. Relax all your muscles, beginning with your feet and progressing up to your face.

4. Breathe through your nose. Become aware of your breathing. As you breathe out, say the word, "one," silently to yourself. Breathe easily and naturally.

5. Continue for ten to twenty minutes. You may open your eyes to

check the time, but do not use an alarm. When you finish, sit quietly for several minutes, at first with your eyes closed and later with your eyes open. Do not stand up for a few minutes.

If you are not in a place where you can sit down and close your eyes, try relaxing by imagining a white light hovering on the top of your head. Breathe in this light deeply so it will fill your whole body all the way to your toes. When you breathe out, imagine breathing out all your problems. Blow out anything that worries you.

EXERCISE

The habit of regular, *comfortable* exercise also has many benefits:

- Improved circulation and increased oxygen in the bloodstream will give you more energy and reduce the feeling of being sluggish and slow.

- Improved circulation to the skin means better nourishment and a more glowing complexion.

- Endorphins, natural pain-relieving substances produced during exercise, will improve mood and promote relaxation.

- As calories are burned, our metabolic rate increases so we keep on burning more calories, even in between periods of exercise. This helps us lose weight and keep it off. Fat instead of muscle is burned for the extra energy, unlike what would occur on a reduced calorie diet without exercise.

- It shapes and firms muscles.

- Most importantly, sensible exercise lowers high blood pressure and our resting heart rate which reduces the risk of heart disease and premature death.

Results of a recent study, published in the *Journal Of The American Medical Association*, showed that people with low levels of physical fitness were twice as likely to die prematurely as people with moderate physical fitness. The researchers found that a brisk thirty to sixty minute walk each day was sufficient. More exercise than this only marginally improved results. The good news is that high impact aerobics, which was the rage of the mid-eighties, is not necessary for keeping fit.

If exercise is fun and enjoyable, and not a form of torture we must force ourselves to endure, we are more likely to do it regularly. Working out at a less frantic pace and lower heart rate is just as effective. We may just need to exercise a little longer. The lower intensity, longer duration exercise will also burn more fat stores.

Even so, it does take some self-control to establish the habit of regular exercise.

'EFFORTLESS' EXERCISE

Sound too good to be true? *Effortless* exercise does exist and consists of electro-muscle stimulation (EMS).

The principle behind EMS is quite simple. When we voluntarily contract a muscle during everyday movement or while exercising, the brain sends a signal similar to a very weak electrical current telling the muscle to contract.

During an EMS session, electrodes in the form of conductive rubber pads are placed on the surface of the skin over the muscles selected to be exercised. When a very weak electronic current is applied through the pads, the signal finds its way through the skin to the muscle and causes it to contract, just as if we had received a signal from the nerve.

First discovered and described by Galvani some 200 years ago, EMS has been used extensively and effectively in physical therapy over the last 30 years to prevent loss of muscle and to stimulate regeneration of muscles in patients who for various reasons have lost muscle tone. For example, following stroke, spinal injury, painful arthritis which inhibits movement due to joint pain, scoliosis and sport injuries. It is also used to manage pain and athletes use EMS as an adjunct to their training and conditioning routines.

EMS has also been shown to be effective in exercising muscles in normal, healthy people. Research by Dr. Charles Godfrey, among others, has demonstrated that the use of EMS builds as much muscle power as does normal exercise.

EMS can be used to re-tone muscles that have lost their conditioning and become lax due to lack of exercise or following pregnancy. The benefits include loss of inches, improving the shape of the figure as a result of tightening, lifting and firming muscles. This is not associated with weight loss unless also accompanied by healthier eating habits.

EMS does not increase muscle bulk, rather it restores muscles to optimal condition. It is therefore very useful not only in restoring body contour but also in preparing muscles for recreational exercise such as snow or water-skiing and scuba diving especially in people who do not exercise regularly.

Starting the conditioning three to four weeks before the holiday will eliminate muscle aching and stiffness which would otherwise occur at the beginning of the holiday due to overstraining muscles not used to exercise. Preparing the muscles in this fashion also reduces the risk of injuring muscles or joints not accustomed to exercise.

An additional benefit of EMS is that it increases circulation without stressing the heart. It therefore does not condition the cardio-vascular system. Active exercise is required for this purpose.

However, EMS does aid lymphatic flow which together with the increase in circulation helps in improving cellulite and clearing toxic waste substances from tissues including skin. This promotes a healthy, glowing complexion.

As with exercise endorphin release is stimulated by EMS. This elevates our mood, gives us a feeling of renewed energy and restores a feeling of well-being.

Used on the face, EMS can also result in gradual tightening of facial muscles. This needs to be performed more gently than on body muscles which respond within 4-8 weeks of vigorous exercise, starting with 35-minute daily treatments until desired improvement is achieved and then reducing to one to two sessions a week as maintenance.

Facial muscles respond better to very gentle application and sessions of shorter duration such as 10-15 minutes once or twice a day for 3-6 months or until optimal improvement is seen and then one to two times a week to maintain the muscle tone.

The most versatile and portable unit available for home or salon use is Ultratone™. The founders of Ultratone™ have had over 30 years of experience in its use worldwide.

SLEEP

Sleep is an essential ingredient for our well-being. Lack of sleep is associated with a number of adverse effects, including less efficient handling of mental tasks and irritability. The effects of sleep loss are cumulative.

It is important not only to get enough sleep but also to stick to a regular sleep routine. Irregular sleeping patterns tend to be associated with feeling groggy and disorientated as well as irritable.

To make up for lost sleep it is best to go to bed earlier the next night rather than staying up late and sleeping in the next morning.

Alcohol and some sleeping tablets can interfere with the brain waves associated with sleep (delta waves), resulting in inadequate rest and symptoms similar to those of lack of regular sleep, including irritability and a lower tolerance for anxiety and stress.

YOGA

Yoga is a form of meditation, body stretching and exercise in which various postures are used to increase self-awareness and elevate consciousness. It is a form of "meditation dance in action" increasing not only spiritual awareness but also producing increased physical and mental well-being.

The yoga postures loosen the joints; they stretch and irrigate the vertebrae, keeping them youthful even late into old age. They promote the free flow of energy throughout the nervous system and assist in the elimination of toxins and poisons from joints and other body parts . . . The postures exert a beneficial pressure on various glands and internal organs, flushing and stimulating them. Even a little bit of this practice can produce astonishing improvements in one's general health.

J. Donald Walters
(Kriyananda)

MEDITATION

Meditation is a means of elevating our consciousness. This requires a two-fold process. The first prerequisite is the cessation of the monkey chatter or self-talk in the beta range of brain wave activity, in which we are almost constantly engaged, even if we may not consciously be aware of it.

Secondly, beta waves are replaced with the consciousness elevating alpha and theta waves as well as the balancing and harmonizing of these brain waves between the right and left sides so that the whole brain is vibrating in unity.

Confirmation that meditation is actually taking place can be obtained by measuring the electrical activity of the brain on an electroencephalogram (EEG) or by experiencing a feeling of contentment, elation or bliss. These pleasant feelings are the result of the release of neurochemicals that have a beneficial effect on our body.

During these states of consciousness we become more receptive to intuitions and inspirations.

What joy awaits discovery in the silence behind the portals of your mind no human tongue can tell.

But you must convince yourself, you must meditate and create that environment.

Paramahansa Yogananda

To learn to meditate effectively in this fashion takes many years of disciplined application. Although it is ultimately the solution to our Western, chaotic, stressed-out mind, it may be a hurdle too large to overcome without some assistance.

For many years now, researchers all over the world, including some of the most reputable institutions such as Princeton University, have been looking for ways to induce the beneficial state that meditation in the Eastern tradition creates in our brain by means of various external devices.

The following is a summary of such devices and their effects on the human brain:

SOUND

For thousands of years, people observed that both light and sound can have a calming, healing, renewing, or exciting effect on our mind, depending on the nature of the sound or light. Sound can be used to shift awareness, to calm or distract the conscious mind and stimulate the brain to vibrate with any particular chosen frequency. That is, specific sounds can entrain the brain waves and thus quickly and easily make the brain vibrate with the desired brain waves, for example, alpha (relaxation) or theta (creativity and meditation).

POWER OF THE SPOKEN WORD

Chapter 1 explained how and why our thoughts have such tremendous power and far-reaching consequences. Imagine then, how much more powerful are the spoken thoughts: our words.

Eastern and other spiritual traditions have long been aware and have employed the power of the spoken word in the form of chants, singing and mantras.

THE EFFECT OF SOUND ON OUR MIND AND BODY

Research shows that the entire body, not just the ear, is sensitive to and responds to sound. Our cells are in a constant state of vibration or resonance. Different parts of our bodies resonate at different frequencies and respond to sound accordingly.

This was confirmed by Dr. William Tiller, Chairman of the Department of Material Science at Stanford University. At the 1976 Conference on the Nature of Reality, he reported, "Each atom and molecule, cell and gland in our body has a characteristic frequency at which it will both absorb and emit (energy)."

The body responds to sound whether positive and life-enhancing or negative and debilitating. Researchers are able to measure responses to sound through muscle testing, biofeedback and biochemical analysis to measure the release of various substances such as endorphins, adrenalin and others.

According to Dr. David E. Bresler in *Free Yourself from Pain,* positive sounds impact the organs and the mind, lower blood pressure (may even break down cholesterol in the blood stream), accelerate body metabolism, minimize fatigue and influence pulse rate among others.

On the other hand, European studies reported in the New York Times show that negative sounds result in abnormal heartbeat, migraines, circulatory ailments, ulcers, more strokes and heart attacks.

Dr. John-David believed that we can experience dramatic transformations in our lives through the use of pure sounds and special frequencies. Research supports this view showing that sound can actually:

- Reduce vulnerability to stress.

- Convert a negative state of mind to positive and thus promote psychological health. Sound has positive effects on depression and anxiety among others.

- Promote faster healing and relief of pain.

- Balance activity in the left and right brain.

- Activate imagination for creative visualization (for many purposes — healing, problem solving, goal setting, etc.).

- Release spiritual energy.

- Liberate creativity by stimulating whole brain activity.

- Correct energy imbalances in the body and mind, and increase energy levels.

Not only does sound have a powerful effect on our physical bodies, certain sound vibrations can balance our brains leading to greater mental capacity and higher levels of performance. When the mind and body are relaxed and our bio-resonance system balanced, the results are effortless action with minimal energy.

According to Dr. Steven Halpern (*Sound Health — The Music and Sounds that Make Us Whole*), "Being in harmony with oneself and the universe" is more than a poetic image. It is resonance or vibrating in our most natural state. The more successful we are in creating environments in which the sound stimuli are in harmony with the vibrational patterns coded into our bodies, the greater our energy, happiness, and health will be.

HEMISPHONICS

Hemisphonics is the latest breakthrough in the sound technology of changing brain waves, called brain wave entrainment. It is used to eliminate the self-sabotaging belief systems which are deeply embedded in our subconscious mind, that is, below the level of our conscious awareness.

Hemisphonics are powerful, positive messages taped within the audible range but mixed with other sounds such as the ocean and soothing music, so that they are not heard consciously, only subconsciously. This reduces the possibility of the conscious mind rejecting these suggestions as they are simply not heard by it. They, thus, bypass the conscious mind, passing straight into the subconscious.

Dynamic Right/Left Brain Programming

Hemisphonics unique technology delivers positive messages to both hemispheres of the brain according to how each best receives and processes information.

The left hemisphere (the rational mind for right-handed people) controls our logic and reason centers. It analyzes the information it receives and organizes it into a logical framework. If the rational mind has had any negative programming in the past it will reject any positive programming.

To sidestep the rational left brain's resistance to positive messages that may conflict with its negative beliefs, Hemisphonics delivers permissive messages such as, "It's okay to succeed." Direct statements could trigger all kinds of negative self-talk from the left brain, such as, "Succeed? I've never succeeded at anything. What makes this time any different?"

The right hemisphere (the creative, intuitive mind) is non-discriminating. It absorbs information without question or analysis. It is here that early childhood messages such as, "You'll never amount to anything," are stored, even though we may not be aware of them. No matter how much we try to re-program negative messages on a conscious level, the imprint may be so deep that negative beliefs will prevail.

Hemisphonics deliver authoritative statements which are readily accepted by our right brain, such as, "I succeed at everything I do," to counteract years of negative programming.

Mirror-Imaging

This is another breakthrough in the Hemisphonics subliminals which increases the effectiveness of the positive affirmations.

Messages to the right brain, the emotional and creative center, are actually recorded in reverse! Scientists believe that the right brain receives language backwards, just as the eyes perceive images upside down and the brain turns them right side up. In fact, some scientists now believe that children first learn language backwards. Recordings of baby-talk gibberish played backwards have revealed intelligible speech. Hemisphonics is the first and only learning program to date to put this astonishing discovery to powerful use.

Hemisphonics powerful messages release negative thoughts, feelings and self-concepts locked in our subconscious and fill our mind with positive, self-affirming thoughts. With less effort, we may be able to change our thinking — and change our life — more quickly.

Hemisphonics can relieve any distorted thinking patterns which can result in stress, fears, and eating disorders, just to mention a few. By correcting distorted thinking for example, excess weight can be lost without diet or exercise.

Subliminal Tapes

These tapes have the positive messages recorded below or underneath the music in the inaudible range of hearing. They are therefore not as effective as the Hemisphonics.

Brainspeak Plus™

These tapes use carefully arranged specific patterns of pure sound to balance the body energy centers, called chakras, by using frequencies that cause vibrations on a cellular level in specific sites in the body and the brain.

They can heighten awareness by increasing the activity of the beneficial brain neurotransmitters.

Some of the tapes in this system combine these pure sounds with positive subliminal messages.

Others use the healing tones of Tibetan bells combined with the music of our own body — specially recorded breathwork, the sounds of the circulatory system, the soothing murmurs in a mother's womb — and the "health" frequencies from Dr. John-David's Sound Library to shift our brain waves into the theta state, where true mind/body healing takes place.

Hypno-Peripheral Processing (HPP)

HPP tapes combine the techniques of Dr. Milton Erickson (father of modern hypnotherapy) and Neuro-Linguistic Programming to effect lasting, dramatic changes in a relatively short period of time. Developed by Dr. Lloyd Glauberman, this is one of the most deeply relaxing and helpful methods of positive change available.

HPP is designed to gently overload a listener's conscious mind by simultaneously feeding a different parable-like story into each ear. Headphones are therefore necessary. This leads to a deep state of relaxation that is ideal for absorbing the positive suggestions on the tapes.

The stories consist of messages that seem to be part of the story, but are actually powerful suggestions to the subconscious. No subliminal messages are used.

LIGHT

Light, like sound has profound physiological and psychological effects on human beings. For thousands of years, light has been known to have a healing influence on the human spirit, mind and body.

Light on its own as well as in combination with sound of a certain frequency, has been found to make the brain vibrate with any chosen brain wave types more easily and speedily.

Several companies have developed "light-sound" machines which are programmed by the use of flickering lights and matching sound to induce brain waves as desired. Alpha waves for relaxation, theta for increased creativity or meditative state, delta for sleep and beta for increased acuity.

There is still some controversy as to what color lights are most beneficial, white, red, green or blue. Most of the light-sound machines are no larger than a walkman and can be used in combination with any of the other technology described here.

BIOFEEDBACK

Biofeedback uses various physiological functions such as blood pressure, heart rate, sweating or brain waves which are measured and reflected on a computer screen so that the individual can learn how to alter these for his/her benefit at will.

Thus biofeedback can be used to learn how to lower blood pressure, heart rate or any other harmful effects of stress.

Most recent advances and applications include programs for teaching how to enter higher levels of consciousness by altering brain waves at will.

It has been observed that once we achieve the desired state with help of the biofeedback, we find it easier to reach the desired states afterward at will, without the biofeedback.

Somewhat like training wheels help children how to bicycle. Once they learn, they no longer need the help of the training wheels. For example, biofeedback could be used to learn to meditate.

CRANIAL ELECTRICAL STIMULATION (CES) DEVICES

Use of these devices is still controversial. Some authorities believe and have demonstrated that these devices can " cure " alcoholism and other drug addictions as well as induce a more harmonious, peaceful state of mind, which is better able to deal with stress. This is done by the use of a very small current which when applied to the scull (behind the ears or on the temples), stimulates the brain to start emitting the more desirable, slower brain waves which result in the production and release of endorphins among possibly other beneficial substances. Endorphins are natural morphine-like substances, which unlike their artificial counterparts are beneficial for the body and mind.

Other authorities believe that not enough is known about the long-term effects of low dose electrical stimulation and therefore do not recommend the use of such devices. Time and further research will tell.

REACH OUT

The Institute for Advancement of Health recently found that people who performed volunteer work regularly for at least two hours every week, were ten times more likely to be in good health compared to those who didn't. Becoming involved in helping others was also associated with a sense of well-being and fewer stress related problems.

CONTINUE GROWING

It would be wonderful if, at the perfect moment, when everything is going well and we are happy, we could stop the changes in our life and continue living in that constant bliss. Apart from being unrealistic, such an existence would eventually result in boredom.

Some people overcome overwhelming odds, while others whose lives are seemingly perfect, are unhappy. The difference is attitude. Our attitude determines whether we perceive a situation as an exciting challenge or as a stressful problem.

So, if you haven't already, open yourself to a new way of thinking and feeling. You have the power to change. Take control of your life and you have found the secret to happiness and a longer and healthier life. And remember, keep a sense of humor and an attitude of gratitude.

CHAPTER

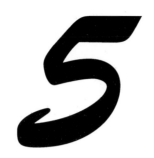

PRODUCTS AND THEIR CORRECT USE

Taking care of our skin requires a life-long commitment that rewards us with looking young, longer.

It is best if skin care starts early — before the first facial wrinkles appear — but don't think it's too late if those first wrinkles have just sounded the alarm.

Taking care of our skin need not be expensive or elaborate. All it takes is a little of our time and some knowledge about how to choose the best skin care products most suited to our complexion.

The cosmetic industry has increased its interaction with dermatologists and established research institutions, and is investing more time and money into research and development of new information and better products.

There is also good news for those concerned about the welfare of animals used in cosmetic testing. Firms are increasingly abandoning animal tests that result in unnecessary suffering, and are searching for alternative testing procedures that do not require the use of animals at all, but rather utilize living cells grown in laboratory cultures.

Areas where new research is likely to result in the development of better cosmetic products include the following:

Quenchers and antioxidants: these are substances that neutralize or eliminate some of the harmful by-products of metabolism.

Research has shown that application of creams containing substances such as vitamin A, E and C can reduce the injury caused by the harmful effects of exposure to ultraviolet (UV) light and other damaging agents such as chemicals. However, it has not been proven that these quenchers or antioxidants applied in creams can prevent skin from aging.

Vitamin E, in particular, may prove to have measurable benefits for the skin. In addition to being used for its therapeutic benefit, vitamin E is added as a preservative.

Vitamin C, which is also an antioxidant, appears to protect against sunburn for as long as three days after application to the skin. A significant portion of vitamin C in the skin is destroyed when exposed to UV light. While vitamin C in the skin does not act as a sunscreen in that it does not directly absorb UV light, it does appear to protect the skin by its anti-inflammatory properties.

Deeper penetrating agents: the development of a new way of delivering beneficial substances, such as sunscreens, moisturizers, antibacterial and antifungal agents and antioxidants, deeper into the skin is also promising. These materials take advantage of the fact that tiny particles like oil micro-droplets are better able to penetrate skin. These tiny particles can be used as carriers for sunscreens, pigments and others, taking them deeper into the skin than they would otherwise be able to penetrate.

Sunscreens: better ways of testing sunscreens are being developed, since reddening of skin after sun exposure may not be the best indicator of damage by UV light. The development of sunscreens that protect more broadly against both UVA and UVB has also led to improved sun protection, as has the development of utilizing natural sunscreens such as titanium dioxide or zinc oxide in a formulation that looks natural and not like the thick, opaque white cream we were used to previously.

Fruit acids, or **alphahydroxy acid (AHA)** compounds: have been used for over 20 years to treat acne. More recently, AHAs have become very popular in the treatment of superficial wrinkles and are discussed in detail in Chapter 7.

Choosing Skin Care Products

This is not easy. In its effort to come up with better products, the cosmetic industry has flooded the market with what seems like an inexhaustible variety of products. It is very difficult to know which products to choose from this vast array.

Some of the influx of new products is due to the increasing competition, with many products having basically the same composition. This makes it even more difficult to decide which products are truly superior.

The ultimate test for the efficacy of a skin care line is how well the products work on your skin.

Unfortunately, in general, skin care companies do not seem to pay much attention to demonstrating efficacy of their products scientifically in volunteers, preferring to use young, beautiful models with blemish-free skin; unlike, for example, the studies on the effects of Retin A and the AHAs which were performed on volunteers with various types of skin as well as those with skin problems.

Over the last thirteen years that I have spent treating skin blemishes and rejuvenating complexions with lasers and other medical procedures, I have been recommending various skin care products.

To my disappointment and that of my patients, I did not find one product line that was problem-free as well as effective.

Over the years, this prompted me to develop a skin care line that would suit all skin types, including very sensitive and sun-damaged skin, and generate the results I and my patients were looking for, while taking a minimum of time from their busy lives.

Most of our skin problems are due to our skin being too dry, too oily or a combination of both. When it is normal, we want to keep it soft, smooth and wrinkle-free for as long as possible.

Solving The Problem Of Dry And Oily Skin

Skin tends to be dry when it produces less of the protective surface oils which form a barrier to the loss of moisture. This tendency is genetically predetermined and aggravated by dry air found in hot and cold climates as well as air conditioned or heated environments.

Removing these precious oils by excessive cleansing can make dry skin even drier. In fact normal skin can become dry under these conditions.

Oily skin tends to produce too much oil. The natural tendency is to try to remove the excess oil with cleansing. However, this produces only temporary relief as removal of the oils stimulates oily skin to produce more to compensate for the excessive loss.

TIME AND SUN DAMAGE MAKE SKIN DRIER

As we get older, our skin produces less and less of the protective and moisturizing fatty surface film making dry skin drier, normal skin dry and oily skin more normal or even dry. The sun accelerates this progression to dryness unless the skin is protected. It also causes damage to the collagen and elastin network which give skin its firmness and elasticity, resulting in wrinkle formation as well as excessive growth of blood vessels known as "broken capillaries."

Sun damage is the major cause of premature, accelerated aging of our skin as well as cancers of the skin. Some of the effects of premature aging can be treated with specific laser techniques as described in Chapter 8.

SKIN CARE

The Basics

Basic skin care involves:
1. Cleansing
2. Moisturizing
3. Exfoliating
4. Protecting from sunlight and other environmental stresses

Cleansing

Cleansers include soap and water, water alone, creams, lotions and liquid cleansers.

Soap And Water

Although soap and water are probably the most effective means of removing real dirt, sweat and especially oils, it is not the ideal.

Removing too much oil may either make your skin too dry if it is already dry or too oily as rebound excessive oil production is stimulated in response to removing too much oil from oily skin. Excessive removal of oils may also result in the skin becoming easily irritated and more susceptible to infection.

The strongest and most drying soaps available are those labelled "deodorant" and abrasive soaps designed for teenage acne. They contain more alkali and are certainly too harsh for dry skin. They may also be too harsh for oily, acne-prone skin.

Milder soaps are often neutral rather than acidic or alkaline and contain more fat or glycerine, which makes them less efficient at removing surface oils and therefore better suited for dry skin and probably also oily skin.

If you have dry skin, use soap only if your skin is dirty enough to need it.

Water

If used excessively on its own, water may, paradoxically, have a drying effect on the skin.

Moderate exposure to water will keep skin plumped up and well moisturized. Excess water, however, will cause the outer layers of skin to become waterlogged. This interferes with the barrier and water-retaining functions of these layers, eventually leading to a loss of water and ultimately drier skin.

Hot water can be even more damaging to the skin, especially if it is already dry. The hotter the water and the longer the exposure, the more of the natural oils are removed.

To protect your skin from water:

- Take short, warm or tepid, showers or baths; avoid too many hot, long baths or showers.

- Avoid strong detergents.

- Use even mild soaps sparingly and only in areas where odors develop.

- Pat your skin dry gently; do not rub vigorously with a rough towel;

this will remove more oils than is necessary or desirable and the friction will irritate your skin.

- While still slightly wet, apply a moisturizer to your skin after bathing. This will replenish the oily layer that has been washed off. Since your skin will absorb some water in the bath or shower, applying the replenishing moisturizer will *trap* this moisture in the skin.

Creams, Lotions And Liquid Cleansers

These are most suited for removing waterproof make-up because make-up is mostly oil-based, rather than water soluble.

If your skin is excessively oily, using creams and lotions alone will make it oilier. You may want to either follow the use of a cream or lotion with mild soap and water, or use a normalizing liquid cleanser such as Amber Essence Clarifying Gentle Cleanser.

If your skin is excessively dry you may just want to use a cream or lotion, or alternate with mild soap and water, water alone, or preferably, Amber Essence Gentle Cleanser as a cream, without lathering it. Always follow cleansing by application of a moisturizer especially if your skin is dry.

Moisturizing

Moisturizers, also known as emollients or lubricants, are cosmetic products that are designed to duplicate the function of the natural oils normally present on our skin.

They reduce the loss of moisture from the skin by depositing a protective seal. They make the outer dead layers of skin softer, more pliable, less prone to cracking, reduce the most superficial, small wrinkles and improve overall texture.

Moisturizers can be either oil-in-water (water-based) or water-in-oil (oil-based) products. Water-based moisturizers are less greasy and lighter than oil-based ones. Oil-based products contain more oil, are thicker and generally provide longer lasting effects. Day creams are more likely to be water-based, whereas night creams are more likely to be oil-based products.

To determine whether a product is more oil or water-based, spread a few drops on your palm. If it disappears without leaving a shiny film, it is likely to be water-based. If it doesn't appear to dry at all, or leaves a shiny surface, it is probably oil-based, unless special ingredients have been added to remove or tone down the shine.

Moisturizers provide a protective barrier against the elements. That is, heat, cold, low humidity and pollution. They assist in sealing in our natural moisture which prevents dehydration.

In the case of oily skin, moisturizers help in balancing our body's production of oil. After repeated cleansing and drying with alcohol-based products, the skin compensates with the production of more oils. This cycle is alleviated by balancing the natural level of oil with a non-oily moisturizer.

If your skin is normal, you may prefer a lotion which deposits a thinner film, but if your skin is dry, you are more likely to benefit from a cream. Lotions contain more water and less oil than do creams. Lotions typically feel non-greasy and appear to be well absorbed by skin. However, the higher water content means that more of the lotion will evaporate, leaving less lubrication on the surface.

Our whole body, not just our face, will benefit from the application of a moisturizer.

The Natural Moisturizing Factor

The presence of a natural skin moisturizing factor has been postulated for many years. A better understanding of how our skin works has shown that the outer layers of skin, previously thought to form only a "husk" made of dead cells, are, in fact, far from inactive. Instead, this layer of skin is a *veritable factory* of oils.

The alternating layers of dead cells and oils also act as a barrier to water loss. Some investigators believe that these oils are part of the *natural moisturizing factor* — the natural mechanism that keeps our skin soft and supple.

Over the last few years a number of cosmetic ingredients have been claimed to achieve the same effects as the natural moisturizing factor. These include urea, lactic and glycolic acids, phospholipids and hyaluronic acid, among others.

All of these, except phospholipids, are able to attract and hold water so that theoretically wherever they go, water follows. The name given to products that attract water is humectants.

Phospholipids are oils that are claimed to resemble and act like the natural oils produced by skin.

Some dermatologists feel their patients benefit from their use, while others do not find them useful. What most dermatologists agree on, is that phospholipids found in cosmetics do not reverse the effects of aging on skin.

In the last few years, creams containing *collagen* or *cross-linked elastin* have been claimed to rejuvenate skin. It is not possible for collagen or elastin in a cream to penetrate into the dermis. Even if they could, they would be attacked and dissolved by the body as any other foreign material.

Exfoliating

Exfoliation refers to the removal of the top excess, thickened, dead cell layer, which accumulates as a result of time and sun damage.

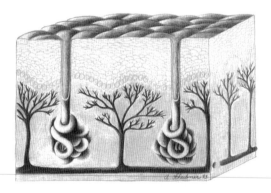

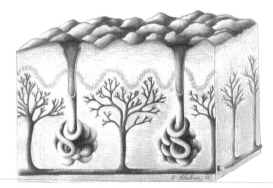

Cross-section of skin in youth.

Cross-section of skin as we age and become more sun-damaged, showing the presence of a thickened top dead cell layer.

Presence of this excess layer contributes to superficial wrinkles. It also prevents the normal extrusion of oils from pores which results in the accumulation and formation of thickened surface plugs, which enlarge pores. These compacted oil plugs turn brown and eventually black by oxidizing upon contact with air, which further accentuates pore size.

Another reason why pores appear to become larger with time is the increased laxity of skin due to loss of collagen and elastin and accumulation of the dry, dead cell layer. This results in the creation of shadows, which give the optical illusion of the pores appearing larger.

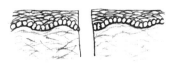

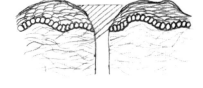

Cross-section of skin when it is smooth and tight.

Cross-section of skin when it is lax. This causes pores to appear larger.

The solution is to exfoliate and tighten skin. This can be done in a number of ways, the most common being the mechanical action of scrubs and the chemical action of light peels.

Exfoliation will not only help remove the top, excess, dead cell layer, but by removal of this layer, stimulates new cell formation in the basal layer. Basal cell turnover can increase as much as fourteen-fold following removal of this top layer.

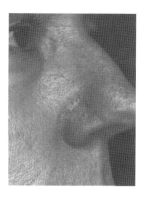

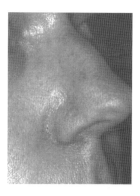

Before

Twelve weeks after using Amber Essence.

The increased cell turnover results in the epidermis becoming "plumped-up," thicker and smoother. In combination with other beneficial ingredients such as the Amber Essence Polishing Scrub and Pore Minimizing Cucumber Toner, the epidermis will also become tighter and the oxidized plugs will be dislodged. Both of these actions have the effect of making pores appear smaller.

Astringents, Toners And Clarifying Lotions

These products are basically the same. Their effect is to tighten skin, temporarily reduce pore size and remove oiliness.

They give a cool, fresh feeling which is caused by the evaporation of the constituents from the skin surface.

If your skin is normal, you can use astringents with an alcohol content of no more than 20 percent. If your skin is oily, the alcohol content may be between 30 and 50 percent.

Those with dry skin should not use astringents containing alcohol as they will have a further drying effect.

These products may be especially useful for acne-prone skin which has excess surface oil. In this case astringents produce a feeling of thoroughly clean skin and make the pores appear smaller. If you have combination skin, use astringents only in the oilier T-zone. However, do not use these products too frequently. Remember, excessive removal of oils leads to rebound oiliness.

Protecting Your Skin From Sunlight

The most important factor in keeping our skin looking young is to protect it from the sun.

Sunlight is the single, most damaging cause of accelerated and premature aging. Sun damage is cumulative. That is, every minute we spend in the sun is credited towards our total skin damage. Exposure during childhood will take its toll in later years when effects of the earlier damage will appear.

We obtain 80 percent of our total life exposure to sunlight before we are eighteen years old.

It is too late for us and the past generations. The damage to our skin in early childhood has been done. But we can take care of our skin from now on and **prevent further damage**. We can also help our children maintain youthful skin by teaching them how to protect themselves from the sun. Sun protection needs to start early in life.

Never assume that you are protected from the sun by simply wearing a hat or sitting under a beach umbrella. UV light reflects off many different surfaces.

It is also important to remember that clouds do not block UV light. We can get sunburned even on a cloudy day.

To prevent excessive UV exposure it is best to avoid sunbathing around midday especially in the height of summer.

Research has shown that how we time our sunbathing will influence the degree of damage to skin immune cells. Least damage results when exposure is limited to fifteen minutes a day for two to three days followed by several days of no exposure and then fifteen minutes a day for another two to three days and so on.

This way of sunbathing will still damage our skin but considerably more damage is produced by daily exposures on consecutive days for two weeks with no rest periods between exposures.

The appearance of **any** tan indicates that some damage has

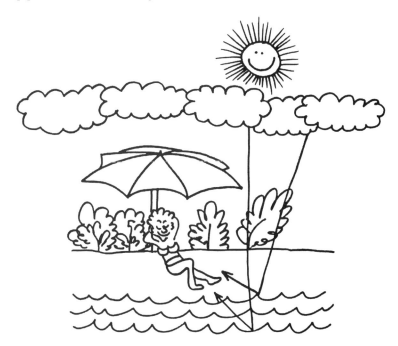

already occurred.

Sun, Medication And Chemicals

There are some oral medications which sensitize the skin to sunlight. If you are using these, you need to avoid direct or prolonged sun exposure as well as protect your skin adequately by wearing sunscreen.

Chemicals in toiletries that might react include oil of bergamot (in fragrances) and biphenyl, a disinfectant.

Some of the drugs capable of causing such reactions include Retin A, antibiotics (tetracycline), tranquilizers, water-loss pills, oral diabetic medications and griseofulvin (an antifungal drug), just to name a few.

If you suspect you are having a reaction to any of these products caused by exposure to the sun, you should discontinue the medication and call your doctor as soon as possible so that alternate medications can be substituted.

Certain chemicals in cosmetics, soaps, deodorants or fragrances, can also cause reactions in some people after exposure to sunlight. The reactions may vary from an itchy rash-like redness to severe sunburn or painful blisters.

Skin Type

There are four skin types based on the skin's response to sunlight. They are different to complexion types:

Type I — never tans
Type II — tans slowly, burns easily
Type III — tans easily, burns occasionally
Type IV — rarely burns

People with skin type I or II can stay in midday, midsummer sun for only five to ten minutes before the first signs of sunburn appear.

Those with skin type III or IV would have to stay two to three times longer before becoming sunburned.

Darker skin is better protected than fair skin. However, even people with very dark skin can become sunburned if exposed long enough. An acquired tan in a person with fair skin is likely to provide very little protection, generally no more than a sunscreen with an SPF of 2 to 3.

Sunscreens

These contain substances that block either UV light A, B, or both. They are rated by measurement of the number of times they increase the exposure time to UVB that would normally result in sunburn of fair, unprotected skin.

This measurement is called the sun protection factor (SPF). A sunscreen of SPF 10, for example, will increase the time it takes for a person with fair skin to burn from five minutes to fifty minutes — ten times more sunlight is required for skin to burn with a sunscreen of SPF 10.

Since these assigned numbers are derived in a laboratory under ideal conditions, swimming, sweating or applying uneven layers of sunscreen, can all adversely affect the time sun protection is provided.

In these circumstances, it is better to apply a water-resistant, or a waterproof sunscreen more thickly and repeatedly so that it remains longer on the skin. It is also advisable to use sunscreen with an SPF of 15.

A water-resistant sunscreen provides protection for about forty minutes of swimming and the waterproof product for eighty minutes.

It is a mistake, though, to think of sunscreens which may not provide total protection from all the harmful effects of the sun, as simply a means of extending time in the sun. IT IS BEST TO LIMIT TOTAL EXPOSURE TO SUNLIGHT AS WELL.

It has been reported by the press that sunscreens of SPF higher than 15 do not provide added protection and may therefore be a waste of money. This is only partly true, since for most people, a sunscreen of SPF 15 should be adequate.

For those with very fair complexion (skin type I or II), or sensitive skin — such as children — SPF factors higher than 15 do provide added protection when spending prolonged periods of time in the sun. However, all sunscreens (with the possible exception of total sunblocks such as zinc oxide or titanium dioxide) allow some UV light to penetrate into the skin.

Some dermatologists agree with the sunscreen manufacturers' recommendations that people with darker complexions (skin types III or IV) need only use sunscreens with SPF of 3 to 5. Others recommend that everyone should use SPF 15 to retard the sun-induced effects of aging.

Besides providing adequate protection for our skin, a sunscreen also needs to be matched to our complexion. People with acne-prone skin need to choose oil-free preparations. Those with dry skin need to choose alcohol-free sunscreens.

Some people may be allergic or sensitive to para-aminobenzoic acid (PABA), until recently one of the most commonly used ingredients in sunscreens. PABA-free preparations are available. These tend to contain less alcohol, are generally less irritating and more suitable for use around the eyes. However, they also tend to be somewhat greasy. If your skin is acne-prone, and you are sensitive to PABA, you may have to try several PABA-free preparations before you find one that suits you.

Amber Essence Moisturizing Protectant SPF 15 was designed specifically to be PABA- and alcohol-free, as well as non-greasy and suitable for all skin types, including sensitive and acne-prone skin.

We also need to remember that lightweight, light-colored, loosely woven clothing may allow a significant amount of sunlight to reach the skin. Dark, tightly woven clothing provides more protection.

Some research has suggested that blocking the sunburn reaction may not block all the damaging effects of UV light. For this reason the SPF may not be the best guide to sun damage, and despite sunscreen protection, exposure to UV light may still result in skin damage such as thickening of the outer skin layers.

Furthermore, there are very few sunscreens that protect against the shortest UV light, UVC. Although the amount of UVC reaching the earth's surface is small, we may find that protection against the C band is also necessary, especially as the depletion of the ozone layer continues.

Unfortunately for the sun lovers **THERE IS NO *SAFE* WAY OF OBTAINING A SUNTAN.**

Artificial Tanning

There are alternatives for those who wish to be tanned. The following are some of the currently available means of tanning other than by natural sunlight.

Tanning salons are not a safe alternative to sunbathing.

Tanning salons: until a few years ago tanning salons were recommended as a safe way of acquiring a tan as the sunlamps emit mostly UV light A. Since then, UVA light has been found to be as damaging as UVB light, if not more so, because of its deeper penetration into skin. It may be even more dangerous because much higher doses of UVA can be tolerated as it causes less redness and discomfort: important signs alerting us to sunburn.

In the United States there are now regulations that control use of sunlamps. In other countries, such as Australia (which has the highest incidence of skin cancer in the world) , there are no enforced regulations controlling sunlamps. Tanning salons cannot be recommended as a safe means of obtaining a tan.

There are four types of artificial tanning preparations, only three of which are safe. None offer any protection against the sun.

Bronzing gels: contain colors which when rubbed on, will last for three to four hours. This is excellent for "tanning" areas such as the face and legs. It would be too expensive and difficult to apply in even layers for a whole body tan.

Quick tans: contain a substance that binds with the epidermis to produce an orange-brown pigment in two to five hours. These can be applied to large areas, although care should be taken to apply an even layer to avoid streaking. The end color will vary from product-to-product and from person-to-person, and usually lasts about one week.

Compared to other products on the market, Amber Essence Self-Tanning Lotion provides a more "brown" tan.

Tan accelerators: contain a protein called tyrosine, which is a precursor to the tanning pigment. In theory, this product is supposed to accelerate pigment production. Whether this, in fact, does happen is still unknown. These products are not approved by the FDA.

Suntan Pills: are no longer available. They consisted of a form of carotene (vitamin A). In addition to possibly being unsafe, they colored the skin an unsightly orange color.

Using Make-Up

How Make-Up Can Enhance Appearance

Many books have been written on the subject of make-up. The purpose of this section is simply to summarize what make-up can do and give some hints on how to use it.

Make-up that is well applied can further enhance certain features and can detract from others. For example, it can cover blemishes or dark circles under the eyes (for those who do not wish to have these medically treated).

Camouflage make-up is used to cover any irregularities in the color of the skin. For example, red birthmarks or the redness after a chemical peel (once the skin has healed) can be hidden or made less obvious. The best way to cover skin discoloration is to choose the opposite color, except for blue, which is best hidden by applying yellow or pink.

To cover green use pink, for red use lime-green and for purple use yellow camouflage make-up. This should be dabbed on just in the area to be covered to reduce the overall thickness of the total make-up.

Foundation is applied next and covers the entire face. The choice of foundation depends on whether your skin is dry, normal or oily. If it is dry use creams, if normal use lotions and if oily use packed powders. It is important not to use a packed powder foundation when skin is dry, as it will dry the skin even more, accentuating creases and wrinkles.

It is also a good idea to choose a foundation that contains a sunscreen. The best way to apply camouflage and foundation make-up is by dabbing it on gently with a firm sponge or with your finger tips.

Enhancement make-up, like lipstick and eye shadow, is the fun part and is applied just under a setting-layer of powder. Enhancement make-up can change your appearance so much, that it is well worthwhile investing money in a consultation by a professional make-up artist. It can give you "painless" cheekbones, large eyes or full lips. In other words, it can make the best of your appearance.

Other than the principles outlined earlier in the chapter, the best way to choose make-up is by trial and error. You can try different kinds by having the cosmetic consultants in the department stores apply them for you. Choose the ones that feel and look best at the end of the day. You may have to try several brands before finding those that best suit you.

Once you find a brand that meets your needs stick to it. Don't change tested and proven products just because new ones may appear better in advertisements, unless you are not entirely satisfied with what you are using.

CHAPTER

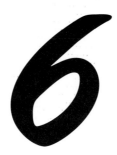

WRINKLES AND CORRECTIVE PROCEDURES

Dissatisfaction with cosmetic procedures most often occurs when people have inappropriate expectations of what a particular procedure can achieve. To avoid disappointment, it is important to know how the aging face can be rejuvenated — there are many different procedures, all suited to correcting specific problems.

Cosmetic procedures are methods used to improve appearance. They include both surgical and non-surgical techniques. Cosmetic surgery is when the skin is surgically cut.

THE ANATOMY OF A WRINKLE

Not All Wrinkles Are The Same

Different types of wrinkles are caused by different kinds of stress and, as a consequence, the treatments vary. There are four basic types of lines or "wrinkles" that develop on the face.

1. The only true wrinkles are the most superficial, fine lines which can run in many directions on the face. These are caused primarily by sun damage and other stresses that dry the skin. Regular use of a good moisturizer can remove or reduce a substantial number of these small lines.

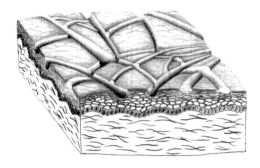

A cross-section of skin showing wrinkles

2. Creases are deeper, individual lines caused by movement, sleep position and sun damage.

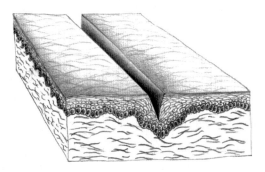

A cross-section of skin showing a crease

3. Folds appear as "elevations" on the skin's surface as a result of gravity and facial movement acting on skin that has lost subcutaneous fat and elasticity. Such loss may be due to age and/or sun damage.

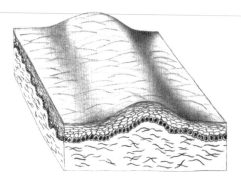

A cross-section of skin showing a fold

4. Furrows are the reverse of folds and are similarly caused — mostly by loss of fat and elastic tissue, as well as facial movements.

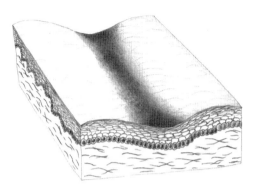

A cross-section of skin showing a furrow

The earliest natural aging event, not caused by sunlight, is loss of skin elasticity and subcutaneous fat. This affects the cheeks first, then spreads to the temples, progressing around the eyes, and finally to the chin and neck.

This process begins earlier in life for those with a family predisposition and those who are thin, that is, those who have reduced fat deposits in the first place.

This may be one reason why many people with rounded, plump faces look younger than those with thin faces. The average age when these changes begin to take effect in a thin person is mid-thirties to forties.

Eventually so much fat may be lost that the redundant skin will hang in loose folds and furrows, the eyes appear sunken, the nose droops and skin around the lips puckers.

CHOOSING A TREATMENT FOR WRINKLES

Superficial, Fine Wrinkles

The easiest of the facial lines to correct are the most superficial, multi-directional wrinkles. Since these are usually caused by sun damage, they are the most preventable, but also the first to appear.

Early on, they respond well to moisturizers, and later to agents that enable the top layers of skin to regenerate, resulting in a tighter, smoother surface. These agents include alphahydroxyacids (AHAs) such as lactic and glycolic acids, Retin A, and light chemical peels.

Creases

The permanent, deeper, individual creases can be filled by injecting materials such as collagen, microlipoinjection of fat, and in some cases, Fibrel.

If there is a lot of redundant skin between the creases, removing the redundant skin and pulling out the creases during face-lift surgery will be successful. However, if there isn't much redundant skin, pulling the skin too tightly during a face-life can result in a mask-like face that looks artificial.

In such a case, a deep chemical peel or dermabrasion might be better than a face-lift. Either of these would produce tightening of the skin and smooth out the creases.

Folds And Furrows

If redundant skin is not present, the lost fat which causes folds and furrows can be replaced. Microlipoinjection is a technique where fat cells from other fat deposits in the body are removed and transplanted to areas on the face.

Individual folds and furrows may also be filled with collagen. If the folds and furrows are not too prominent, chemical peels may also be beneficial. However, all of these procedures are less likely to be as dramatic or as long-lasting as a face-lift or other surgical alternatives. If the problem is excess fat creating folds, liposuction may help.

In time, gravity will further exacerbate the problem of loosely hanging skin and eventually produce jowls, droopy eyelids, double chins and even longer and floppy earlobes.

The surgical procedures invented to reverse the effects of gravity and return to normal the important cosmetic features, have been some of the most successful in cosmetic surgery.

These surgical procedures are designed primarily to correct the effects of redundant skin. When they are used to improve superficial sun damage, fine wrinkles or lines caused by movement, the results can be disappointing.

CHAPTER

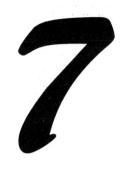

ALL ABOUT COSMETIC PROCEDURES

This chapter deals with the various cosmetic procedures available today and what can be expected in terms of indications, technique, healing time, improvement and complications. Although it describes many side-effects and complications, it is not meant to dissuade you from undergoing cosmetic surgery, merely to make you as fully informed and prepared as possible.

ALPHAHYDROXY ACIDS

What Are Alphahydroxy Acids

Discovered to have many beneficial effects on our skin in the early '70s, alphahydroxy acids (AHAs) are derived from fruits such as apples, oranges, grapes, as well as from other foods like cultured milk (lactic acid) and sugar cane (glycolic acid).

How Alphahydroxy Acids Work

When applied to the surface of skin, these compounds have several beneficial effects on the skin, depending on their concentration. At low concentrations (2% to 12%), AHAs reduce adhesion of cells in the dead, dry skin cell layer, allowing it to exfoliate faster and preventing its accumulation. This has the effect of reducing dry, scaly, wrinkled and blotchy appearance of skin, making it appear smoother, softer, less wrinkled, and more even-toned.

The exfoliating effect also helps pores empty their contents, preventing the formation of black heads and pustules and thus improves acne.

At high concentrations (30% to 70%), AHAs have more penetrating and more profound effects resulting in the epidermis sloughing off so that new regenerated epidermis grows in. This results in the skin not only looking less wrinkled, but also containing fewer sun-damaged cells.

AHAs can also stimulate collagen and elastin formation in the dermis which helps the elimination of wrinkles, making skin appear smoother and tighter.

AHAs appear to be less irritating than Retin A. They also appear not to be associated with some of the problems of Retin A, such as the appearance of permanent "broken capillaries," observed to occur following prolonged use of Retin A.

The high concentrations of AHAs should be applied only by experienced professionals. AHAs are left to work on the skin for less than one to several minutes before they are washed off thoroughly to inactivate them.

The areas will remain red for several hours and depending on the exact concentration and length of application, may or may not peel over the next three to four days. Healing is completed within five to ten days, depending on the concentration of the AHAs.

RETIN A

What Is Retin A

Retin A is a medication. It is a vitamin A derivative and has been found to reverse many of the detrimental effects of ultraviolet light on the skin. It was first used more than thirty years ago by researchers in Pennsylvania, who found it had many beneficial effects on acne. Since then, the product has been refined to the currently available formulation known as Retin A.

Retin A exerts measurable changes in the epidermis and dermis of skin, which can be long-lasting.

How Retin A Works

In the epidermis, Retin A promotes early loss of dead cells from the surface. This makes the skin feel smoother, softer and more sensitive to touch. However, it can also leave the skin more sensitive to irritation from some perfumes, moisturizers and sunscreens, as well as, more susceptible to sunburn and sun damage. It is important to use a non-irritating moisturizer and a good sunscreen every day. Itchiness and dryness develop if moisturizers are not adequately applied.

Retin A also increases the turnover of epidermal cells and normalizes pre-cancerous cells. Some pre-malignant lesions, known as actinic keratoses, may disappear with treatment. Deeper or more extensive skin cancers will have to be removed surgically.

Retin A disperses pigment, making the skin look less mottled, less yellow and lighter in color. Age spots may lighten, but usually require additional treatments (see Chapter 8). Melanoma, a dangerous cancer of pigment cells requires surgical excision.

In the dermis, Retin A stimulates the repair and production of new collagen and elastin which makes skin stronger, less wrinkled and can accelerate wound repair. Growth of new blood vessels is also stimulated. Retin A does not remove broken capillaries. In fact, it has recently been reported to promote the appearance of permanent skin redness by stimulating the growth of blood vessels.

All of the effects of Retin A are greatest on the most sun-damaged skin. Thus, the mild irritation and increased sensitivity noticed in the first three months are simply the normal results of Retin A and show that it is working. The irritation settles once most of the repair has occurred.

It is possible to aggravate these side-effects. To avoid irritation it is best to avoid the following:

- Heat and sweating immediately after application.

- Sun exposure without protection.

- Excessive sun exposure even with protection.

- Occlusion by watches or jewelry.

- Application in the deep skin creases around the nose, or too close to the eyes.

Studies have shown that everyone will notice some improvement after three months.

Despite this, Retin A is not a panacea for all types of wrinkles. Lax, sagging, deeply wrinkled, yellowish skin with excessive folds is beyond Retin A repair. Also, if you are a sun lover, you ought to consider the advantages versus disadvantages of using Retin A.

How To Use Retin A

Retin A is a **medication** and should be used under the supervision of a physician familiar with it.

People with fair skin can start using it in their early 20's as a skin cancer preventive measure, **but only if they are willing to forego sunbathing and use sunscreens whenever in the sun, even while driving to work.**

Those not willing to live without a tan, should not use Retin A. It makes the skin more susceptible to sunburn and thus possibly increases the risk of skin cancers.

People with olive complexions who are prepared to stay out of the sun can start later — between thirty and forty years of age. Their skin is naturally better protected.

If your skin is thin and generally sensitive, start applying the lowest concentration of 0.01 percent Retin A once or twice a week at night. Gradually, increase application to once a day and eventually if tolerated — that is, if your skin does not become too irritated, red, itchy or sore — to twice a day. It is important to apply only a small amount, and keep it away from the eyes, deep creases of the nose and corners of the mouth. Your skin should be thoroughly dry before you apply Retin A.

Daily application should be continued for a minimum of twelve months and then twice a week, probably forever, as maintenance treatment.

Pregnant women, nursing mothers and those with hypersensitivity reactions such as eczema and allergic reactions to vitamin A should not use Retin A.

RENOVA

What Is Renova

Renova is the trade name of another retinoic acid topical product which has been submitted to the FDA for approval in the treatment of wrinkles.

How It Works

Being a retinoic acid derivative, Renova works in a fashion similar to Retin A. We will no doubt hear more about this product when it becomes available.

LIGHT OR FRESHENING CHEMICAL PEELS

What Are Peels And How They Are Used

Various chemicals can be used to peel away the outer layers of the skin. The result is most consistent and predictable when used to treat sun damage. After treating sun damage with chemical peeling some or all of the sun-damaged tissue is replaced. The top layer of the dermis is renewed and normal epidermis with none, or fewer, pre-cancerous skin cells, grows back.

The effects of a peel will depend on the depth of penetration.

Peels can be light, medium or deep. How deep a peel extends, depends on the type and concentration of the peeling agent, how long it is allowed to remain in contact with the skin, whether oil was removed from the surface prior to its application, whether Retin A was used for several weeks or months or occlusive dressings were applied afterwards. Both Retin A and occlusive dressings increase the depth of penetration. Light peels are quicker, less painful and heal faster than deep peels.

Peels will also tighten skin, partially correcting the effects of gravity, as well as, some movement-related lines. These effects are only temporary, whereas the repair of sun damage seems to be permanent unless sun exposure is continued.

How A Light Peel Works

A light peel destroys the outer layers of skin. When the new epidermis grows back it has a smoother surface with fewer or no pre-cancerous cells.

A light peel will improve only the small, superficial wrinkles, including those around the eyes where the skin is especially fine. Very light peels can be used on the neck, chest, arms and hands. Medium and deep peels should only be used on the face, as there is a considerably higher risk of scarring other places on the body, especially the neck.

The chemical agents used for light peels include plant enzymes, such as papaya or pineapple, extracts of pancreatic (digestive) enzymes and low concentrations of various acids. The most commonly used acids are 20 percent trichloroacetic acid and various concentrations of lactic, glycolic or salicylic acids.

How A Light Peel Is Applied

The face is first washed with a cleanser such as soap and water and wiped with alcohol. The peeling agent is then painted on the skin using a cotton-tipped applicator. Within thirty to sixty seconds the skin begins to burn, like a sunburn. Although the discomfort experienced is directly related to the strength of the peeling agent, it varies tremendously from person to person, based on individual pain tolerance.

The burning sensation is relieved by fanning the face with cold air or ice packs, and, regardless of its severity, it subsides completely within a few minutes.

Afterwards the skin may feel tight. It will be red for several hours and then may appear dry for three to four days. The top layers begin to peel off at about this time, either as tiny flakes or as whole sheets, like sunburn, depending on the depth of the peel.

The peeling is complete in seven to fourteen days.

Although the new skin is tighter after the peeling is finished, it will continue to improve over the next few weeks or even months. The effects of a light peel may last for four to twelve months.

Repeated or deeper peels may have more long-lasting effects by stimulating new collagen formation in the dermis.

Possible Side-Effects And Complications

There are usually very few complications after light peels, especially if only the mildest concentrations of agents are used.

However, they are by no means unheard of. If complications do occur, they are generally temporary and less troublesome than those following deeper peels.

Uncommonly, some people do experience a darkening or lightening of skin for a period of several months after a light peel. The darkening usually fades but can be removed more rapidly with the use of bleaching agents. Routinely using sunscreens (at least SPF 15) every day as well as staying out of the sun, especially in the first two weeks after a peel, may help avoid this complication.

The opposite effect, loss of pigment or whitening of skin, is rare with light peels. This complication is more common after deeper peels. It may be permanent, but can be corrected by laser treatment or tattooing pigment into the skin (see Chapter 8 and 9).

Hypertrophic or raised scarring caused by light peels is even more rare than pigmentation problems.

Unlike deep peels, it appears that light peels can be repeated many times without obvious permanent damage. This is possible because the wound is superficial and appears to heal completely.

However, there are some pre-existing conditions that may slow healing, even following a light peel. These include previous X-ray treatment (a common treatment for severe acne some thirty years ago) and prolonged use of cortisone.

MEDIUM AND DEEP CHEMICAL PEELS

What They Are And How They Are Used

Medium and deep chemical peels have more profound effects than light peels and are used to treat moderate and severe sun damage, respectively. The effects on skin are as described for light peels. The changes are long-lasting enough to be considered permanent.

Because high concentrations of chemical agents are used, the treatments are too painful to be tolerated without medications. Most doctors will use intramuscular or intravenous pain medication either in their office or in a hospital.

The agent most commonly used for deeper peels is phenol or carbolic acid. When used cautiously by an experienced professional, phenol is a very effective peeling agent. It can, however, cause complications during the procedure. The most serious complication is irregularities in heartbeat which can be life-threatening and is thought to have been responsible for several unexpected deaths during deep phenol peeling. This toxic effect is related to the speed of phenol application. It should take a minimum of one hour to peel the whole face. The patient's heartbeat is constantly monitored in order to prevent this reaction. If there is a change in the heart rhythm, the speed of application can be adjusted, avoiding any serious problems.

Interestingly, it is not the highest concentrations of phenol that necessarily produce the most serious toxicity. Phenol diluted with water, in a 50 percent solution, appears to be more toxic and produces a deeper peel than the full-strength phenol which is an 88 percent solution.

Removing the oil from the surface of the skin and pre-treating with Retin A has to be taken into account when considering the concentration of phenol to be used. Both result in deeper absorption of the peeling agent. Olive oil applied to the skin, on the other hand, may diminish its penetration and hence reduce the depth of peel and the potential toxicity.

Other agents used for deep peels include higher concentrations of the agents used for light peels, as well as, pure alcohol.

How Medium And Deep Peels Are Applied

As with light peels, the face is first washed with soap and water and then wiped with alcohol. With medium and deep peels pain medication is given before the peeling agent is applied. The pain from a deep peel begins twenty to forty minutes after application, and may last for four to six hours before abruptly stopping.

The next day, the face is mildly to severely swollen, especially around the eyes. In fact, it may not be possible to open the eyes for several hours each morning.

Swelling and pain can be prevented or significantly reduced when Diapulse technology is applied (see Chapter 8).

The swelling generally subsides in three to four days, but can take longer if the skin is delicate or sensitive. It is also helpful to elevate the head of the bed by putting something like telephone books under the head end of the mattress or using several pillows and by applying cold pressure packs.

Some doctors also use cortisone, either by intravenous injection or as tablets, given during the procedure or for a day or two before and for up to a week after the procedure. Provided there are no medical contraindications such as diabetes, ulcers or high blood pressure, the dose of cortisone received in one week will not lead to any long-term complications.

However, the Diapulse is a safe and more effective alternative.

Since the treated areas may ooze, and when allowed to dry form crusts, some doctors recommend washing the face with soap and water two to three times a day to prevent crusting.

This is followed by application of an antibiotic ointment for several days and later by an anti-inflammatory cream.

Some crusts will form despite washing, but these flake off, generally in one to two weeks.

The softer the crusts or scabs are kept, the less irritating and less thick they become, and the lesser the chance of infection. After the crusts flake off, the skin is smooth but remains sensitive and red for at least another month.

The deeper the peel, the longer the healing time. Healing is generally not complete for about six months, unless Diapulse is used, in which case it will heal faster.

Make-up can be carefully applied after the scabs fall off and new skin has grown over the chemically peeled area. Even light make-up will generally cover any redness still visible. Make-up should not be applied too early as it may disrupt the newly grown, delicate skin and delay healing.

Possible Side-Effects And Complications

It is best to be prepared for possible complications, as the incidence with medium and deep peels is fairly high. Fortunately, most can be treated with medication and will disappear with time.

Loss of pigment can be considered a normal side-effect, rather than a complication of phenol peels. It almost always occurs. It may not become apparent until three to six months after treatment.

Phenol peels are therefore best reserved for those with fair, sun-damaged complexions who do not intend to continue to tan. Phenol is not suitable for those with olive or dark skin. This recommendation may change in the future as patent-registered techniques have recently been developed (see Chapter 8). These may stimulate hypopigmented skin, that is skin that has lost pigment (for example, following a phenol peel), to re-pigment. However, the degree of re-pigmentation or whether it occurs every time cannot be predicted with certainty.

Even if the skin is fair, a noticeable line may develop between the phenol treated face and the neck. The neck may be considerably darker due to sun damage, but cannot be peeled with phenol as it is likely to scar. Feathering the peel carefully from the face to just under the jaw where the line between the peeled face and untouched neck would be less visible, will help but may not avoid the problem if the skin on the neck is permanently discolored due to sun damage.

This discoloration may be due to broken capillaries or excess brown pigment and may fortunately be treated with specific laser techniques for the former (see Chapter 8) or very light peels for the latter.

Skin on the neck is finer and more sensitive than on the face. Light peels may be used with caution on the neck, but they will not remove the broken capillaries. Only specific laser techniques can do that.

Amber Essence Moisture Radiance and Pore Minimizing Cucumber Toner have been observed to reduce the discoloration presumably by a *calming* effect on the capillaries.

An increase in pigment can also develop, especially following medium deep peels which can irritate rather than destroy pigment cells, resulting in excess production of pigment. This pigmentation is usually blotchy rather than uniformly darker and appears two to six weeks after treatment. It can be prevented or at least reduced by avoiding the sun altogether, if possible, for the first six to eight weeks. If this is not possible, routinely applying sunscreen with SPF of at least 15 after the first week and for a minimum of three to six months, will help.

The redness that normally follows a deep or medium peel may be accompanied by itching and burning. This usually lasts a few weeks and can be relieved by aspirin or Diapulse treatment.

More rarely, the patchy redness may persist for up to six months. It is difficult to cover with make-up and is accentuated by the normal blushing response to embarrassment, anger or heat. Fortunately, the redness usually eventually subsides without treatment.

Infections of the peeled skin can cause much more serious problems, including scarring, if they are not treated adequately, or in time. Fortunately, even though infections occur fairly commonly, particularly with deeper peels, permanent scarring is infrequent and can also be treated with specific laser techniques, developed recently (see Chapter 8).

Infections can be prevented by carefully following the doctor's instructions, and by seeing the doctor, or his or her staff, at the first signs of infection — excessive redness, oozing, swelling or pain.

If scarring does occur it is usually confined to smaller areas on the upper lip and around the jaw. Most of the time, early treatment with cortisone cream, injections or laser treatment will prevent a thick scar. Other types of scars can include a patchy loss of the normal skin markings. This can develop when more than one deep peel has been applied. Only light peels can be repeated safely.

It is important to let the doctor know if you have ever had a cold sore, which is caused by the herpes virus. This virus is often activated by the peel and can spread to the whole peeled area. To avoid this, you are treated with specific medication prior to and after the peel.

Another rare complication is the development of swelling around the vocal cords, which may develop in the first twenty-four hours, but apparently only in heavy smokers. This is a potentially life-threatening complication that needs immediate medical attention.

Within the medical profession there are doctors who routinely perform medium and deep peels and are enthusiastic about the procedure. There are also doctors who are opposed to it. Medium and deep peels can produce excellent results; but, they are also associated with a significant risk of complications, including scarring, and should be performed only by doctors well trained and experienced in this procedure.

DERMABRASION

What Is Dermabrasion And How It Is Used

Dermabrasion is a sanding technique first used by dermatologists and plastic surgeons to correct acne scarring. It utilizes a fast-rotating wire brush or a drum with a diamond coating to sand the skin. It is the mechanical equivalent of medium and deep peels but requires even more expertise to administer. The level of skill required may explain why some physicians are even less enthusiastic about dermabrasion then they are about chemical peels.

One of the reasons for this may be that dermabrasion is not always performed for the right reasons.

Dermabrasion is the procedure of choice for shallow, superficial scarring, particularly from acne and particularly in people with thick, oily skin.

Abrading thick skin is easier than abrading thin skin because there is less chance of sanding too deep. Sanding may also reduce the oiliness and improve any residual acne. Chemical peels do not work as well on thick, oily skin. The chemicals do not penetrate as well.

Abrasion for correction of sun damage is appropriate only when there are other reasons for dermabrasion, such as acne scarring.

As a general rule, men with sun damage who have thick skin are more suitable for dermabrasion, while women with sun damage who have thin skin are more suitable for a peel.

Excess pigmentation caused by birth control pills or pregnancy may lighten or even disappear with abrasion (see Chapter 8 for more detail on this condition).

In addition to acne scarring, dermabrasion is beneficial for other types of scars including some resulting from trauma or surgery. It can remove the ridges at the edge of skin grafts as well as reduce elevated hair transplants.

The effects of a dermabrasion are similar to that of peels. The outer skin layers are mechanically removed to a variety of depths, depending on the severity of scarring to be treated. When the new skin grows back, it is tighter and smoother. If skin cancers (actinic keratoses) were present, they too may be removed.

How Dermabrasion Is Performed

Since dermabrasion involves bleeding, it is essential to tell your physician about any medications you are taking, such as aspirin or vitamin E, as they may increase bleeding.

Birth control pills can cause water retention in the skin, making it possible to abrade the skin more easily and quickly, and therefore, more deeply than may be desirable. The pill may also increase the risk of the skin becoming darkly pigmented after abrasion.

Those with a history of cold sores should be pre-treated with antiviral medication and those with heart valve disease with antibiotics.

Because the procedure involves possible handling of blood by the doctor and his staff, you may be requested to have hepatitis B and AIDS or HIV antibody tests before surgery.

Dermabrasion is not recommended for AIDS patients because of the difficulty in dealing with possible infections.

Some physicians believe a small test spot abrasion is appropriate to determine how the skin is going to react. It can also demonstrate to the patient what one can expect from the procedure. Since different parts of the face react differently, it is difficult to predict how the whole face will react, so testing is not uniformly performed.

The procedure begins with the skin being cleansed with soap and water or alcohol. A wire brush or diamond fraise is used to evenly sand away the skin to the required depth. This can range from a superficial wound, all the way to the equivalent of a deep peel.

The stinging or burning sensation is too painful to tolerate without pain medication. Most doctors use intravenous sedation and a freezing spray that has an anesthetic effect and makes the skin easier to dermabrade. The majority of doctors perform dermabrasion in their offices.

As soon as the abrasion is completed, a dressing is applied to stop any stinging, reduce the discomfort, collect the ooze, protect the abraded skin from infection, and speed the healing.

The next day, the face is washed in the shower, gently, with soap and water. Any crusting that may have formed is removed and the dressing is changed. Contrary to what one would expect this is not very painful and can be quite refreshing.

After patting the areas dry, an antibiotic ointment is applied. A new dressing can then be used for one more day or the skin can be left uncovered. Some doctors prefer the dressing to be reapplied daily for one to two weeks.

After the face is washed an ointment is applied twice a day for four to five days. After this the ointment is switched to an antibiotic cream (which is thinner than ointment) with or without cortisone, depending on the doctor's advice.

It takes about one to two weeks for new skin to grow over the abraded areas, depending on the depth of the abrasion. If an area was purposely abraded deeply to remove deeper scars, it will take longer to heal. Infection and excessive movement (like smiling, laughing and chewing) also prolong the healing time.

The redness generally disappears faster than after a deep peel, and only rarely lasts up to six months.

It is important to carefully watch any areas that are healing slowly as this may be an indication of possible scarring. For this reason, most doctors will want to see you several times during the first two to six weeks or ask you to report any persistent redness, swelling or pain. Immediate treatment may prevent scarring.

It is absolutely essential to avoid sun exposure for at least three to six months after dermabrasion. If your skin is sensitive, even one inadvertent, mild sun exposure (five minutes of midday sun for fair skin!) can result in excess pigmentation. It may take six to eight weeks for this pigment to first appear.

In general, the earlier the excess pigment appears, the more likely it is to disappear in less than six months; the later it appears, the more likely it is to be permanent and require further treatment to remove it.

Possible Side-Effects And Complications

As with medium and deep phenol peels, loss of pigment can be regarded as a side-effect rather than a complication. It can occur in as many as 50 percent of all dermabrasions; while that following deep phenol peels occurs in almost all cases.

An increase in pigmentation can also result in a blotchy discoloration. It can be prevented, or at least reduced, by avoiding the sun in the first three to six months. Reabrading or peeling the blotchy areas that persist can reduce the discoloration. Bleaching creams may also be used. They are more effective if used early.

Milia are small pinpoint white spots that appear in almost all patients. They usually disappear without any consequences. Some doctors have found they can be prevented by scrubbing the face immediately after an abrasion with gauze and saline.

Active acne may flare-up in some patients, but usually resolves quickly.

Scarring is obviously the most serious complication. It can occur in areas where the skin was more deeply abraded, or the depth was extended by infection, irritation or repeated movement.

Skin that was previously treated with X-rays also risks being scarred as does skin in diabetics who are malnourished, patients who have other predisposing diseases or patients who have taken Acutane.

It has been suggested that the acne medication, Acutane (isotretinoin), may increase the risk of hypertrophic — red, raised thick — scarring. It has been advised to delay dermabrasion for six to twelve months after discontinuing Acutane.

This does not appear to be the case with superficial laser treatments which have been performed without any problems within weeks of discontinuing Acutane.

Scars can occur suddenly, often between six weeks and three months, most commonly around the lips and jaw. It is best to treat them early and continue careful follow-up by your doctor.

LASERABRASION

What Is Laserabrasion And How It Is Used

Laserabrasion is a recent addition to the available cosmetic procedures. Basically, it is a dermabrasion performed using carbon dioxide or argon lasers. Lasers have been in use for over thirty years. However, this is a new application. Because it is such a recent development, the risks of treatment, complications and long-term follow-up for this procedure are not yet available. In the United States, only a handful of doctors perform this procedure.

Laserabrasion involves using lasers to heat the skin enough to burn or destroy the outer layers to be removed. The burning may increase the risk of scarring unless the treated area is limited and the professional operating the laser is experienced in this particular use.

FILLERS

What Are Fillers And How They Are Used

Fillers are substances which are injected into the skin to elevate individual creases and furrows. Fillers are not suitable for the correction of multiple facial lines that are too numerous, or when gravity and loss of supportive tissues has caused prominent redundant skin folds.

Many filler substances have been used over the years. Some, like paraffin, have been discarded. Others, like silicone in breast implants or microdroplet injections, have been recently withdrawn, pending further investigation into the reported complications.

Collagen, Fibrel and fat transplantation are still used today. All have slightly different properties which make them best suited to different applications.

COLLAGEN

What Is Collagen And How It Is Used

Collagen is the most widely used filler product. It is made of purified calf skin collagen and comes in three forms. Its use was pioneered by the Beverly Hills dermatologist, Arnold Klein, M.D., who has the most extensive experience in its use, having injected over 20,000 patients since the late '70s.

Zyderm I contains more water and less collagen than **Zyderm II**. It is easier to inject and is best suited for the finest or most superficial wrinkles. It is also used to make lips fuller. (This use is not FDA approved). **Zyderm II** is injected deeper into the skin and is most effective for treatment of furrows.

Collagen can be used for the correction of lines and scars anywhere on the body. It has been injected for many years under corns on feet to relieve pressure. Deep, ice-pick acne scars and small punched-out acne scars do not respond well to collagen injections. Since all currently available collagen is made from animal protein, our body utilizes it and it disappears. However, the injected collagen acts as a scaffold for cellular and vascular ingrowth which may result in some more permanent correction.

Zyplast has been designed to last longer and is used to elevate the deeper lines and furrows. It is more resistant to breakdown, more resilient under physical pressure and retains more water.

In addition to this, Zyplast has the added advantage of stimulating production of the patient's own collagen adjacent to the implant site. The amount of new collagen produced varies from person to person.

Unfortunately, Zyplast is not suitable for correcting small, superficial wrinkles. It is only used for deep furrows.

Most of the correction obtained from injected collagen (both Zyderm and Zyplast) disappears within six to twenty-four months, depending on the skill of the professional injecting it and individual patient variation. Eventually it moves out of the skin into the subcutaneous tissue, except over bony prominences and in scars, where the implant may be trapped by the underlying bone or the thicker scar tissue. The recommended total volume of Zyderm I injected in any twelve-month period is 30 cc and Zyderm II is 15 cc. Collagen comes in 1 cc syringes.

How Collagen Injections Are Performed

Anyone considering collagen injections must first have a skin test to make sure they are not allergic to it. About 3 percent of the population may be allergic. In those who are allergic, almost 90 percent of the positive reactions become apparent in the first three days after the test. A small number become positive during the first four weeks.

A positive reaction consists of a red, itchy, swollen spot at the injection site. It may take several weeks or months to go away. Even when the first skin test is negative, there is a 1.5 to 2 percent chance that an allergic reaction to the injected collagen may still develop, which shows up in the first few weeks. This has influenced some doctors to perform two tests. The first test is done on the forearm. If this is negative, another test patch is done on the other forearm and just inside the hairline on the face four weeks later. If this is negative in another four weeks, the center of the face is injected as necessary.

It is not unusual for some doctors to only wait two weeks before doing the full procedure (90% of allergic reactions take place within the first 3 days).They also may not routinely do double testing. If results of the first test are negative and there is no questionable history or possible previous reaction to collagen, they may forego the second test.

Most people will tolerate collagen injections, even in the most sensitive areas around the mouth and nose without any pain medication. Ice packs may be applied before the injections to reduce discomfort.

A topical anesthetic cream which requires thirty to sixty minutes to work is available. This is simply Novocaine (lidocaine) applied in a cream form instead of injection. A pharmacy can make this preparation with a doctor's prescription. An injection may also be used to numb the nerves around the mouth and nose.

The smallest disposable needle is generally used to inject the collagen. Any discomfort experienced, other than the needle prick which is minimal in most sites, is caused by the local anesthetic liquid which comes mixed with the collagen. After a few minutes, the injected areas become numb.

Because lines on the face are more prominent when sitting or standing, most doctors will do the collagen injections while the patient is sitting or reclining on a couch.

When Zyderm is used, the wrinkles are over-corrected. That is, more collagen is injected than is needed. This is because a significant portion of Zyderm is water, and the water is absorbed during the first day. Only one to two-thirds of the injected volume remains.

Possible Side-Effects And Complications

There are four possible complications after collagen injections:

1. allergic reactions
2. swelling
3. mechanical problems, and, more recently,
4. the question of possible autoimmune diseases such as polymyositis and dermatomyositis, which are chronic progressive and some-

times fatal inflammatory disorders. To date, there is no evidence that these disorders are higher in patients who have had collagen injections in comparison to the general population.

Allergic reactions

Allergic reactions can occur even after a negative skin test. Double testing will reduce, but not prevent, the chances of missing a person's allergy to collagen.

If reactions do occur, they are always localized to the injection sites, and will appear red or swollen and occasionally become itchy. They are worst during the first few weeks and gradually settle over the next few months.

The reactions are rarely severe. Only a very small percentage of the 3% of patients who are allergic develop generalized complaints such as joint and muscle pain, headache, itch, rash or swelling.

Allergic reactions are less common with Zyplast than with Zyderm, but are more likely to occur over bony prominences, such as the forehead and cheek bones. Injections may also be associated with the recurrence of herpes simplex (cold sores).

There is no specific treatment for allergic reactions. They will usually subside in time.

Swelling

Swelling is seen in about 1 percent of people treated with collagen. This occurs at the injected sites and in about half the cases, redness appears with the swelling. This reaction can last intermittently up to three years.

The swelling can be triggered by exercise, sun exposure, menstruation, or consumption of alcohol, cocaine or beef. The skin sites appear perfectly normal between flare-ups. Different sites can flare-up at different times.

An intermittent swelling reaction does not mean that discontinuation of collagen injections is necessary, but a skin test should be repeated to ensure that this is not a true allergic reaction.

Mechanical

Mechanical problems include bruising at the injection site, overcorrection, a yellowish discoloration from collagen injected too superficially or into skin that is very thin, like under the eyes and more rarely scars. All of these reactions, except scars, will disappear with time and without treatment. Scars resulting from collagen injections can be treated with lasers (See Chapter 8).

Massaging may help to speed up resolution of overcorrection by pushing the collagen deeper into the skin. Some doctors will always massage immediately after the injection to make the implant less visible from the beginning.

There have been reports of a small number of people developing skin damage at the injection site which on occasions healed with small, flat, depressed scars. This may have been due to accidentally injecting blood vessels, and appeared to occur more commonly with Zyplast injected into superficial wrinkles, such as those on the forehead where Zyderm would be a better choice.

Infections have also occurred but are not serious and typically resolve spontaneously or with antibiotics.

Autoimmune Diseases

> *Some physicians have reported that patients developed polymyosites (PM) dermatomyositis (DM), which are chronic progressive, sometimes fatal inflammatory disorders, and other connective tissue diseases after receiving collagen injections, even though they never had these diseases before. FDA is investigating whether there is a cause-and-effect relationship between having collagen treatments and later developing PM/DM or similar diseases.*

FDA Backgrounder

To date, there is no evidence that these disorders are higher in patients who have had collagen injections in comparison to the general population.

Contraindication

A complete medical history is required before collagen is administered to rule out any contraindications to the injection of collagen. These include: history of autoimmune diseases such as rheumatoid arthritis, lupus (SLE), scleroderma or myositis (an inflammatory condition involving muscles). Patients with a history of severe allergic reactions such as anaphylactic (life threatening) shock should also abstain. Those who are allergic to lidocaine are also non-candidates for injections. The effects on infants, children or pregnant women are not yet known.

Collagen should never be injected into inflamed or already-infected areas. Never have injections into breasts that have implants or into bones, tendons, ligaments, muscles or blood vessels.

Hylan Gel

Hylan gel is a new substance currently under investigation for FDA approval to be injected, like collagen, as a filler substance to correct wrinkles. It is a form of hyaluronic acid which is a significant component of our skin.

Derived from a number of sources both plant and animal, hyaluronic acid is currently a very useful ingredient in moisturizers, active as a humectant. (A humectant is a substance that attracts water.) Hyaluronic acid draws one thousand times its weight of water into the skin.

Initial studies with hylan gel appear to be promising. One of its advantages may be a more long lasting effect. Since it is still derived from animal or plant sources, the incidence of allergic reactions or other side effects remains to be seen.

Silicone

What Is Silicone And How It Is Used

To date, all the different techniques and products containing silicone have been labeled with the one name "silicone." Not all silicone products are the same and not all appear to be associated with the adverse effects reported in the lay and medical press. As a result, a useful product, the "injectable-grade silicone" has been withdrawn from the market. Even prior to the FDA prohibition of silicone use, only a handful of doctors who felt very strongly about the superior ability of silicone to treat certain facial lines used the product. Some were injecting tiny drops of silicone to correct scars and reduce wrinkles for over twenty years with excellent results.

Because of the enormous expense that would be involved in repeating the basic experimental work that the FDA has requested, for a product that is not patentable, it is unlikely that silicone will be FDA-approved in the near future, which is a prerequisite for its use, unless the FDA accepts studies already performed.

The American Academy of Dermatology and the American Society for Dermatologic Surgery have undertaken a joint task to review all information available on injectable liquid silicone. There is some hope, depending on the findings of the committee that this may influence the final word on injectable silicone.

The advantage of silicone over the other fillers was its performance. The tiny injected drops of silicone eventually were surrounded by natural collagen which prevented the silicone from moving or being digested. The injected silicone appeared to be permanent and also appeared to *grow* a little as new native collagen was deposited around each tiny silicone droplet. This is why silicone injected sites were under-corrected. If large volumes of silicone were injected, the silicone was reported to move to other parts of the body, including the liver.

It must be stressed that the success of silicone injections depends on use of the proper technique and the highest quality silicone. If too much silicone was injected, adverse reactions included movement of the silicone to other parts of the body, inflammation, rusty-brown or pink discoloration of the surrounding tissues, and formation of granulomas (lumpy areas of inflamed tissue). These types of complications on the face can now be treated with specific laser techniques (see Chapter 8). Those on the body resulting from large amounts of silicone injected to enlarge breasts or other soft body tissues to change body contour are too extensive for any significant correction at this time unless the injected sites are not too large.

Silicone was used to elevate soft, depressed and distensible scars. It could also be used for wide or deep furrows such as the smile line or the grooves under the eyes or around the lips, neck creases, and furrows due to loss of fat on the back of the hands. Silicone was also useful for correcting the small irregularities that sometimes develop after cosmetic surgery, especially on the nose, and when permanent fullness of the lip was desired.

There was also a great deal of experience using silicone for correcting foot problems such as corns. The injection of silicone for feet was the only FDA-approved use.

How Silicone Injections Were Performed

There are no known allergies to silicone so a skin test was not required.

The injection of silicone was almost painless. All that was felt was the needle prick and some sensation of pressure as silicone liquid was injected. The smallest available disposable needle was used to inject minute amounts of silicone.

Some doctors massaged the site afterwards to further break up the droplets.

Improvement was noticed within a short period of time. Several visits at four to ten week intervals were necessary to completely correct a depression. Only small amounts of silicone could be injected at each session. Deep furrows required four to six injection sessions for complete correction. As with other treatments for movement-related lines, maintenance injections were required every few years.

Possible Side-Effects And Complications

The incidence of adverse reactions following the microdroplet technique using injectable-grade silicone was reported to be very low.

Temporary redness could develop at the injection site in about one-fifth of the patients. It lasted anywhere from hours to three days, without leaving any remaining marks on the skin.

A few patients have been reported to develop long-lasting dusky redness. Some doctors think this reaction is the result of adulterated "silicone" or from injecting too much silicone. This can also be treated with specific laser techniques (see Chapter 8). Cortisone may also be used but the response is slow, and cortisone injections have the added risk of possibly causing loss of too much tissue resulting in uneven depressions of the injected skin.

More rarely, darker pigmentation, blue-brown in color, may have occurred at the injection site. This appeared to be more common when silicone was injected to fill defects after surgery on the nose.

Itching, bruising and infection were infrequent and resolved without treatment. These can be expected when anything is injected into the skin.

It was easier to over-correct with silicone than with other fillers because it becomes larger in time, whereas the others are absorbed and become smaller. This problem could be avoided by injecting only tiny amounts and no more frequently than once every four to ten weeks.

Unlike these relatively minor complications, many more serious complications have been reported following the injection of massive amounts of adulterated silicone directly into breast tissue, or from leaking silicone breast implants. Some of these complications include arthritis, hardening (fibrosis) of the breast tissue and migration of the silicone resulting in the distorted appearance of the breasts. More recently a rare condition called scleroderma and other immune system related diseases have been reported in association with leaking silicone implants. With scleroderma, the skin and possibly other organs become tight and hard, eventually resulting in a mask-like face (smiling becomes difficult) and many internal complications of a similar nature (hardening of organs).

Silicone is no longer injected. There do appear to be problems associated with the presence of large quantities of free silicone in the body.

Silicone And Breast Implants

It is well known that the breast implants used many years ago would *bleed* or leak silicone which was associated with the arthritis reported. Since then, *low-bleed* breast implants have been developed which are lined with material that is less permeable to silicone.

However, recent reports in the press are raising questions about the safety of some of the coated implants. The most controversial appear to be those coated with polyurethane foam. No-one knows what happens to this chemical when it eventually breaks down in the body. Long-term studies and more research on the effects of silicone and other substances used in implants are needed to determine the safety of these products. Meanwhile, if you are considering having breast implants, ask plenty of questions.

To help you, the following is information on breast implants quoted from the FDA Backgrounder published in August of 1991:

Important Information On Breast Implants

Approximately 2 million American women have breast implants, either for reconstruction after breast cancer surgery or to enlarge or reshape the breasts. Most of these women have not experienced serious side effects. But like all medical devices, breast implants do pose some risks. Therefore, a woman who is considering having breast implants must decide, with her doctor's help, whether she is willing to accept these risks in order to achieve the expected improvement in her appearance.

Before a woman can make that decision, she must understand what the risks are. To help women gain this understanding, the U.S. Food and Drug Administration has prepared the following information. It briefly summarizes what is known and not known about the risks of breast implants, and what the FDA is doing to resolve the unanswered questions. This information applies to women who are considering having implants, as well as those who already have them. Some of the possible risks are not completely understood right now, but as more information becomes available, the FDA will make it known to the public.

For a woman considering breast implants, reading the following information should be just the first step in finding out about the risks. It is very important that she know this by discussing the possible risks with her doctor. He or she can provide more comprehensive and specific information and can explain how the risks apply to her particular case. Some women have found it helpful to ask the doctor for a copy of the implant package insert, which lists the possible adverse effects in some detail.

The surgeon can also provide information on the different types of implants available, as well as possibilities for surgical alternatives that do not require implants.

1. What kind of breast implants are available?

The most common types are described below. Each has its own advantages and drawbacks. Your physician is in the best position to describe these to you.

• *Silicone gel-filled.* This is the most common type of implant. It is a silicone rubber envelope filled with soft, silicone gel that feels like very thick jelly. The envelope may have either a smooth or textured surface.

• *Saline-filled.* This is a silicone rubber envelope filled during surgery with sterile salt water (saline solution).

• *Double lumen.* This implant has two silicone rubber envelopes, one inside the other. One is filled with silicone gel by the manufacturer. The other is filled during surgery with a small amount of saline solution. This permits the surgeon to adjust the size.

2. What are the health risks associated with silicone gel-filled implants?

The adverse effects associated with silicone gel-filled breast implants can be divided into two categories: **known effects**, which are experienced by some women and are clearly associated with these devices, and **possible effects**, which might exist but have not been proven.

The most common of the **known** effects is hardening of the scar tissue that normally forms around the implant. (This is called capsular contracture.) This can sometimes cause pain, hardening of the breast, or changes in its appearance. Calcium deposits can also form in surrounding tissue, and this too can cause pain and hardening. There is also the possibility that an implant may rupture, allowing the gel filling to be released into surrounding tissue. If the problems are severe, the implants may have to be removed permanently.

Other known effects include temporary or permanent changes in nipple or breast sensation due to the surgery.

The **possible** effects are chiefly related to silicone gel that may escape from the implant and reach distant parts of the body. This can happen if the implant ruptures, or if tiny amounts of silicone leak or "sweat" through an intact implant. (This is also referred to as "gel bleed".)

It has been suggested that even the very small amounts of silicone that "sweat" through the implant could cause certain autoimmune (connective tissue) diseases, such as lupus, scleroderma, and rheumatoid arthritis in some women. Some physicians have reported that a few of their patients have developed arthritis-like diseases after receiving breast implants. **But there is no conclusive evidence at present that women with breast implants have an increased risk of developing arthritis-like diseases or other auto-immune diseases — that is, women with breast implants who have developed such diseases may have done so regardless of their implants.** *

Questions have also been raised about whether silicone in breast implants can increase the risk of cancer or pose a risk to unborn babies. Although these possibilities cannot be ruled out, there is no evidence at present that women with breast implants or their unborn babies are at increased risk. Studies to prove or disprove a link between silicone and cancer or risks to unborn babies are now in progress (A study several years ago linked implanted silicone to cancer in rats, but the tumors produced were not the type that occurs commonly in humans).

3. How about the risks of the saline-filled implants?

Some of the known effects, including hardening of the scar tissue and calcium deposit formation, occur with both the gel-filled and the saline-filled implants. Rupture of the implant may be more likely with the saline-filled type, so women with these implants should be especially careful to avoid trauma to the breast such as might occur from falls or very active sports. When a saline-filled implant ruptures, it is more likely to deflate quickly, requiring surgical removal.

On the other hand, rupture or leakage of a saline-filled implant results in the release of salt water, which is not foreign to the body, whereas rupture of a silicone gel-filled implant releases silicone gel, a foreign substance. This may have a bearing on the unanswered questions about silicone breast implants: Since the saline-filled implants do not have the silicone gel, they are probably even less likely to increase the risk of autoimmune diseases or cancer. But since both types of

---

* Bold type added.

implants have the silicone rubber envelope, such effects cannot be totally ruled out, even for the saline-filled implants.

4. Will implants interfere with results of mammography exams? Will having a mammogram cause my implants to rupture?

Both the silicone gel-filled and saline-filled implants can interfere with the detection of early breast cancer because they can "hide" suspicious lesions in the breast and because having implants makes mammography more difficult to perform. Also, any calcium deposits formed in the scar tissue around the implant may interfere with interpreting the mammogram. And, since the breast is compressed during mammography, it is possible for an implant to rupture. (This may be more likely for the saline-filled type.) These problems can be reduced by making sure the mammography facility you select is accredited by the American College of Radiology (ACR) and by asking if the personnel at the facility are experienced in performing mammography on women with implants. Discuss the selection of an accredited facility with your physician. You can also call your local chapter of the American Cancer Society or the National Cancer Information toll-free hot line at 1-800-4-Cancer for a list of ACR-accredited facilities in your area.

Before your mammography exam, it is important to tell the technologist that you have implants. She should take special care when compressing the breast. Also, an experienced technologist knows how to push the implant away from the breast tissue to get the best possible views of the tissue.

5. What about polyurethane-coated implants? Do these pose a special risk?

About 10 percent of women with silicone gel-filled implants have a special type that is coated with polyurethane foam. The coating is intended to reduce the risk of capsular contracture. The FDA is concerned about the polyurethane-coated implants because polyurethane can chemically break down to release very small amounts of a substance called TDA, which can cause cancer in animals. But it is not known whether there is a risk of cancer from TDA in women with this type of implant. Until the risk, if any, to women with polyurethane-coated implants is determined, the manufacturer has agreed to stop shipping these implants and has asked physicians to stop implanting them. In the meantime, FDA is requiring the manufacturer to conduct further research in this area, analyzing blood, urine and breast milk for TDA, using a representative sample of implant patients. In order to resume marketing polyurethane-coated implants, the manufacturer will have to provide FDA with data demonstrating their safety and effectiveness.

6. What about a woman who already has polyurethane-coated breast implants?

The cancer risk, if any, is likely to be very small. If the polyurethane foam coating on these implants were to chemically break down in the body at the same rate as in laboratory experiments, the lifetime cancer risk for a woman with two implants would probably be less than 1 in a million, assuming she retained the implants for 35 years. If the polyurethane were to completely break down — which is unlikely to occur — the risk would be about 1 in 12,000.

Based on these risk estimates, there is insufficient evidence at present to support having polyurethane-coated breast implants surgically removed because of concerns about cancer.

7. Is there a risk to a nursing infant from the polyurethane coating?

At this point, there has been one report that a trace amount of TDA from polyurethane may have been found in 1 out of 3 samples of breast milk from one woman. This single report does not constitute adequate evidence that TDA enters a woman's breast milk or that there is any risk to a nursing infant. However, FDA is requiring the manufacturer of the polyurethane-coated implants to conduct further studies on breast milk. Studies will also be conducted on TDA levels in blood and urine.

8. Does the silicone gel itself pose a risk to a nursing infant?

Although the possibility that silicone might cause cancer or autoimmune diseases in humans cannot be ruled out, there is no evidence at present that this is the case. It is therefore unlikely that the trace amounts of silicone that might enter the breast milk of a woman with implants could increase the risk of her child's developing these diseases.

9. How can I know which implants I have?

Women who already have implants can find out from their implant-

ing surgeons or from hospital records, if available. Those planning on having implants can ask their surgeons for a photocopy of the "sticker" that identifies the implant by brand name, type, product number, manufacturer, and date of implant.

10. How long will the implants last? Are they permanent or will I have to have them replaced after a certain length of time?

The exact life span of an implant is unknown and varies from woman to woman. Implants last for many years in some women and have to be replaced more frequently in others.

11. Should women concerned about the possible long-term risks of breast implants have them removed?

The two greatest concerns to most women with implants are cancer and autoimmune diseases. **But at this time there is no proven association between breast implants and development of these diseases. The scant information that is currently available on possible risks does not warrant removing the implants,** *especially considering that any surgical procedure carries a risk of its own. Nonetheless, a woman who is concerned about the possible risks or who is experiencing problems she feels are associated with her implants should consult with her doctor to decide what is best in her case.*

12. Is one brand or type of breast implant safer than another?

Some doctors prefer a particular type because they have experienced more success with it in some respects — for example, in avoiding certain adverse effects. But until FDA evaluates the safety and effectiveness of the implants, it will not be known for certain whether one brand or model is safer than another.

13. Where can women report problems they think are caused by their implants?

Problems related to breast implants can be reported to the implanting physician and the implant manufacturer (if known). Problems can also be reported to FDA by calling (1-800) 638-6725. Within Maryland, call collect at (1-301) 881-0256. (Please note that these numbers are for problem reporting purposes only; they are not information hot lines.) Include the following information, if known:

- *manufacturer's name*
- *product brand name and catalog number*

- *product style, size, and lot number*
- *date of implant surgery*
- *date of problem*
- *nature of the problem*
- *name and address of surgeon and facility*
    where surgery was performed
- *(optional) your name, address and telephone*
    numbers

The above information was quoted directly from the *FDA Backgrounder.*

FIBREL

What Is Fibrel And How It Is Used

Fibrel is a filler made of pork-derived (porcine) gelatin protein, which was approved by the FDA in 1988.

Fibrel is mixed with a portion of the patient's own blood before being injected into the skin. In the skin, it forms a sponge-like material which is eventually replaced by natural collagen and blood vessels.

The early experience suggests that Fibrel may be better for treating depressed scars rather than wrinkles. Zyderm and Zyplast are still the best for treatment of wrinkles; that is, folds, furrows and creases.

Fibrel appears to last longer than Zyderm collagen. It has been reported that as many as 85 percent of the corrections were maintained for one year and 79 percent for two years.

About 2 percent of the population appear to be allergic to porcine collagen. A skin test is performed four weeks prior to treatment. Since transient redness and swelling almost always occur, a reaction is only considered positive if the redness lasts more than two to four days.

People allergic to Fibrel may not be allergic to Zyderm and vice versa.

How Fibrel Injection Is Performed

The technique used to inject Fibrel is quite different to that for collagen and silicone. With Fibrel, **some tissue injury is necessary to produce the desired response.**

A pocket is created under the scar or furrow, which is filled with the implant material. This is too painful for most people to tolerate without a numbing injection.

Overcorrection by 50-100 percent is necessary. Once the mixture is injected, it is molded into place under the scar or furrow by finger massage. Only one or two treatments are necessary in most cases to correct depressed scars.

Possible Side-Effects And Complications

Redness, swelling and nodules are quite common at the treatment sites. The redness and swelling usually subside over the first week or two. The nodules which are dusky red may persist for a month and only rarely leave a permanent dark mark.

The time it takes for the redness and swelling to disappear may present problems cosmetically. Zyderm and Zyplast can make you look great immediately, but Fibrel takes at least two weeks.

Fibrel has been reported to result in sloughs when injected into creases between the eyebrows. That is, the skin overlying the injected Fibrel breaks down forming an ulcer, and is lost, which can result in a scar.

Some people report an immediate feeling of nausea, faintness or a headache. These reactions are possible whenever anything is injected into the skin and may not have been related to Fibrel itself.

MICROLIPOINJECTION

What Is Microlipoinjection And How It Is Used

Microlipoinjection is the transplantation of fat cells, usually from the thighs, abdomen, buttocks or knee pads to areas which have lost their fat deposits. For example, on the face, making the fold between the nose and corner of the lips excessively prominent, or back of the hands, which results in the veins appearing quite large. Loss of fat may be caused by age, disease, trauma or cortisone.

Fat transplantation is not new. It was first used in the nineteenth century. The current technique, however, is quite new. It was first proposed by Pierre Fournier in 1976. There is still much to be learned, especially about critical factors required for fat cell survival at the new sites. The techniques are still subject to controversy.

Fat transplantation has a very specific application: to replace fat where it has been lost. It is not suitable for superficial wrinkles (where chemical peels or dermabrasion may be more appropriate), or creases (where other fillers are better suited), and only a face-lift will take care of excess skin.

Loss of fat is a normal part of the aging process. It affects the whole face. Smile lines deepen, the eyes appear to sink, the cheeks hollow, the chin recedes, the skin above the lip puckers and loses its sharp border. Only fat transplantation will initially correct this loss of fat on the face. In time, the loss of fat is accompanied by the appearance of redundant skin, which is best corrected with cosmetic surgery.

How Microlipoinjection Is Performed

Both the withdrawal and injection sites are first cleansed with an antiseptic and then wiped with alcohol. Cold packs may be applied to reduce pain and blood loss. Diluted numbing solution is injected into the site from which fat cells are to be withdrawn.

The Fournier method involves removing fat cells by gently withdrawing them into a syringe, with a fairly large needle. Others remove fat with suction machines.

The fat cells are washed after they have been removed and then injected into the recipient area with an over-correction of at least 100 percent. Not all the fat cells will survive. The new fat is molded with finger pressure.

Injection of fat into the face is both quicker and less painful than removing the fat. The recipient area can be numbed, but this is done with as little distortion of the furrows as possible. For example, by injecting the numbing solution around the nerves that provide sensation to the area to be injected.

Some doctors apply a dressing to help stabilize the new cells. Posttreatment care varies and may include cold compresses, oral antibiotics, and minimal facial movement.

The cosmetic results vary. Frequently there is only a 30-40 percent retention of the new cells. In some patients there may be no retention. For those in whom the fat cells survive, correction is usually long-term and in half of these it may be permanent.

When the area is only partly corrected, the transplant procedure can be repeated until a satisfactory result is obtained. The failure of one graft doesn't mean that the next will not be successful.

Possible Side-Effects And Complications

To date, there seem to be few complications. They include bruising at both the donor and recipient sites, swelling that subsides in time and possible asymmetry when more of the fat cells survive than anticipated (one side of the face is uneven compared to the other side). If this doesn't improve in time, it can be corrected by either adding to the opposite side or taking away some of the fatty tissue.

BOTOX

What Is Botox And How It Is Used

The use of Botox has recently appeared as another means of combating creases caused by movement such as frown and smile lines.

Botox is an extract of the highly toxic poison produced by bacteria that cause botulism. The chief danger of botulism is that it causes muscle paralysis which when extensive can cause death due to paralysis of muscles necessary for breathing.

Small amounts of this substance injected with delicate precision can be used to paralyze specific small muscles and thus prevent the skin creasing caused by these muscles. To produce longer lasting paralysis, repeat injections of Botox are required.

The effects have been reported to last from several to eighteen months. Longer lasting results may be due to possible muscle damage.

Possible Side-Effects And Complications

Excess weakness of the injected facial muscles can cause restricted movement; for example, droopy eyebrows or eyelids. Muscle damage may also occur.

As with all new treatments, time is required to adequately assess all the possible benefits as well as any deleterious effects.

FACE-LIFTS

What Is A Face-Lift

The face-lift is a cosmetic surgical procedure best suited to the removal of redundant skin and tightening of the underlying tissues. Used appropriately, it can dramatically create a more youthful face.

Face-lifting is not new. It was first performed in Europe at the beginning of this century. At first, only the skin was pulled tighter. However, as more and more skin was being removed the incidence of widely stretched scars and loss of skin increased to an unacceptably high level. The next development was to loosen skin by undermining or parting it at the level of the fat layer, which allowed skin from the center of the face to be moved instead of just being pulled at the edge. This was still not the perfect answer because eventually, the skin would begin to droop again.

In 1976, two plastic surgeons, Mitz and Peyronie, demonstrated that there is a continuous sheet of strong connective tissue attached to the underlying muscle that extends from the side of the nose to the front of the ear and down the neck muscles. It is called the Superficial Musculo-Aponeurotic System or SMAS for short.

Lifting and sewing this lining in a higher position on the cheekbone where it used to be, before time and gravity did its damage, will provide a longer lasting result and a truly rejuvenated appearance as the underlying muscles are also tightened and restored to their younger position.

The most recent refinement in face-lifting has been the addition of liposuction and cheek and chin implants. Liposuction allows fat to be removed from areas where there is too much, such as the neck and jaw, improving results of face-lifts.

Particular face-lift techniques vary from doctor to doctor. Generally, the face is *lifted* in two directions: *up*, which tightens muscles on the neck, under the jaw and chin; and *sideways* which tightens the cheek muscles and anchors those around the jaw, chin and neck.

Despite the improvements in face-lifting procedures the main smile line (the groove that runs from the nose to the corner of the lips) remains the most difficult of the face lines to correct. Face-lifts almost never correct the upper half of this groove.

If this is an area that is particularly bothersome, it can be improved with collagen or microlipoinjection. To try and smooth this groove surgically may result in a face that looks too tight, or even nerve damage.

How Face-Lifts Are Performed

A face-lift is a long procedure that some doctors prefer to perform with an assistant. Depending on the extent and length of the procedure, it may be performed with local anesthesia, general or intravenous sedation.

The face-lift incision is generally placed in front of the ear, as close to the ear opening (even inside) as possible to reduce its visibility. It then slopes behind the ear into the hairline. If the earlobe is droopy or floppy, it is reshaped. The skin is then undermined or parted at the fat layer and pulled up sideways. The excess skin is cut off and the remaining skin stitched in front of the ears. In time, the tightness produced by this operation will lessen. However, a face that has been "lifted" almost always looks more youthful years later, even if maintenance surgery is not repeated. If you want to continue looking as youthful as after the first face lift, a maintenance procedure will be required in two to five years.

In the second operation the face can be pulled much tighter by lifting and sewing the scar tissue that formed as a result of the first operation — a normal, and in fact, desirable effect. The second face-lift may produce a tighter, smoother face than the first.

After the surgery, a firm dressing consisting of a complete head wrap is applied. Facial movement will be limited because of swelling, discomfort and possible muscle weakness and numbness. The swelling will resolve in seven to fourteen days, any discomfort will disappear even earlier. The numbness may last several months.

If the Diapulse is used in the first few days after surgery, healing occurs twice as fast and there is significantly less swelling, bruising and, therefore, discomfort. Any numbness also resolves faster.

Stitches are sequentially removed. The stitches in front of the ear are removed by the fourth day, and those in the temple and nape of the neck, where the tension is greatest, are left in for about ten to twelve days. The stitches are replaced by small pieces of tape called Steristrips which hold the skin tightly together. Some doctors recommend using the Steristrips for several weeks to prevent stretching or widening of the incision line. This may make the line less visible. Specific laser treatments will also help induce the elimination of scars even when these have been present for a long time.

Possible Side-Effects And Complications

The overall reported rate of complications varies from 4 to 20 percent and includes bleeding, infection, skin loss, hair loss, asymmetry and nerve damage. Although complications can occur even in the most experienced hands, it is probably true that the more skilled, and experienced plastic surgeons have fewer complications.

It is essential to tell your doctor if you are taking aspirin or other medications that interfere with blood clotting. However, bleeding can occur in anyone. If the swelling becomes worse in the first few days after surgery, you should notify your doctor as this may indicate a fresh bleed. If the accumulation of blood is large the surgeon may drain it to avoid further problems such as skin loss.

Where the skin is thinner or pulled very tightly, it may not receive adequate blood supply. It may then slough or be lost, usually in the first seven to ten days after surgery. Fortunately, this happens only very infrequently, and when it does, is usually limited to small areas. If any visible scarring remains, this also can be treated with specific laser techniques (see Chapter 8).

It has been established that smoking may cause sloughing. Some doctors will not do a face-lift on heavy smokers. Others insist that the patient stop smoking for several weeks before and after surgery.

Nerve damage is usually only temporary and resolves itself within a few weeks or months. Weakness of the lower lip is more common when muscle work and liposuction are done to lift muscles under the jaw and to remove jowls or a double chin.

Permanent nerve injury is uncommon and occurs when more extensive surgery is done under the SMAS, close to the center of the face, in an attempt to smooth the nose-lip groove.

Numbness of the earlobe also occurs infrequently. This may eventually resolve but can take months or even years.

As many as 15 percent of face-lift patients may experience temporary or permanent hair loss in the temple, nape of the neck or in front of the ear where the incision is made.

Facial asymmetry can occur and, if it is noticeable, may require a second procedure to correct. If it is not that prominent it may improve with time. Trimming and reshaping the earlobes is done carefully so that they are both even.

Infection is rare after a face-lift and responds readily to antibiotics. On rare occasions, broken capillaries which may have been present but not very noticeable may become more prominent. These may subside in time or, if they do not, they can be treated with lasers.

EYELID SURGERY

What Is Eyelid Surgery And What It Can Do

The medical term for eyelid surgery is blepharoplasty.

Eyelid surgery does marvels when there is redundant skin around the eyes. If there is sagging elsewhere on the face, improving only the eyes can make the face look unbalanced; that is, the eyes may look youthful in an older face.

The eyelid skin can appear droopy not only when there is too much skin, but also if the eyebrow droops due to a lax brow.

One way of determining whether excess folds around the eyes are due to excess eyelid skin or to a droopy brow is to lift the eyebrow up over the bony prominence above the eye, where it should normally be. If nearly all of the redundant eyelid skin disappears, the problem is with the eyebrow and not the eyelid. In this case, some doctors would recommend a brow-lift. Others would still prefer eyelid surgery.

Dark circles under the eyes are usually not removed by lid surgery.

They may, however, improve by reduction of the shadows resulting from redundant skin folds under the eyes, that can exaggerate the dark circles. The procedure will not correct sun-damaged skin, which is better treated with chemical peeling or certain laser techniques (see Chapter 8).

How Eyelid Surgery Is Performed

Most surgeons who perform eyelid surgery, but are not ophthalmologists, recommend a full eye examination by an ophthalmologist prior to surgery. Eyes that are relatively dry can be operated on, but the amount of skin removed from both the upper and lower lids is less than when the patient does not have dry eyes. If too much skin is removed the eyelids will not close completely, and the eyes may become even more dry.

If a brow-lift is being performed as well, it is usually done first, followed by the upper eyelid and lastly the lower eyelid surgery. This is to avoid removing too much skin.

Eyelid surgery can remove baggy skin, excess fold of fat or a combination of both.

The excess fat can be removed through a cut on the inside of the lower eyelid. A cut on the outside isn't necessary. However, even if it were required, eyelid skin heals so well that the suture lines are nearly invisible.

The surgery can be performed using either local or general anesthesia. Afterwards the eyes will be swollen and discomfort may be experienced for the first few days, although this is usually minimal. Bruising may be present for seven to fourteen days. Dressings aren't usually necessary, but it is advisable to sleep on several pillows or elevate the head of the bed (for example, by placing a telephone book under the head end of the mattress) and apply ice to help reduce swelling. Diapulse applied in the first few days following surgery will also reduce swelling and pain and accelerate healing.

Possible Side-Effects And Complications

As with face-lifts, bleeding can occur, so it is essential to tell your doctor if you are taking aspirin or other blood anti-clotting medication.

If the bleeding is noticeable in the first twelve hours, the lids should be examined by the surgeon. If there is sufficient evidence of bleeding, the blood should be drained and bleeding stopped. It is essential to let your doctor know immediately if you feel you may be bleeding. If the blood is not drained and re-absorbs on its own, the collection of blood can create an unevenness in the overlying skin.

Another possible complication is dry eyes. The most common cause of dry eyes is the inability to close the lids during sleep. This can happen during the first few days after surgery when the eyelids are still swollen. Taping the eyes closed can help avoid the problem.

In time, the skin may loosen. If it doesn't loosen sufficiently, a skin graft may be required to correct the problem.

It is possible that eyes are irregular in shape before surgery. This may have been camouflaged by redundant skin but will become more noticeable after surgery. It can be corrected by further surgery.

Rarely, drooping of the upper lid can occur. It is caused by damage to the muscle that elevates the eyelid. Excessive swelling and bleeding can distend the muscle fibers causing such damage. It usually corrects itself within several weeks. If it doesn't, surgical repair of the muscle may be required.

Drooping of the lower eyelid may lead to the white of the eye showing. It may also cause eye dryness if the lids do not close completely. The drooping can be caused by the removal of too much skin from the lower eyelid, or from a scar that develops because of excessive bleeding or hematoma. If the downward pull is quite pronounced, or if it interferes with normal eye function, the lower lid can be repaired with a skin graft.

Infection is extremely rare and usually responds to antibiotics. The development of an infection severe enough to cause an abscess around the eye has been reported in one of the many hundreds of thousands of procedures performed to date.

Nerve damage is also rare and usually resolves in time, although it may sometimes take several years.

BROW-LIFTS

What Is A Brow-Lift And What It Can Do

Lifting of the brow can be beneficial for people whose brow droops due to lax or excess skin.

This operation may not be possible if the hairline and forehead are already high as the lift may further raise the forehead height. The skin can be removed from the forehead itself, but this may leave an undesirable scar.

How long a brow-lift will provide improvement depends on how heavy the forehead skin is. If it is heavy, it tends to fall again within a few years and requires further surgery.

How Brow-Lifts Are Performed

There are various ways of elevating the forehead skin. The skin can be removed well into the hairline, from the middle of the forehead (just outside or inside the hairline), and just above the eyebrow.

If excess skin is the only problem, the redundant skin is removed. If there are forehead grooves due to muscle wrinkling, the muscle can also be tightened or cut so that it is no longer able to cause frowning.

If deemed advisable, Botox to paralyze the muscles causing frowning may be injected. A dressing is applied and the swelling and healing are similar to that following a face-lift or blepharoplasty.

Possible Side-Effects And Complications

Infections are rare and excessive bleeding is less common than following other surgery involving looser tissues like the neck or cheeks.

Prolonged and even permanent numbness and itching of the scalp behind the incision line can occur.

Removal of skin directly from the forehead by excision in front of the hairline rather than by lifting it through undermining via an incision in the hairline, can result in visible scars on the forehead. Fortunately these can be treated using specific laser techniques (see Chapter 8).

The results can also be asymmetrical but this can be improved by a second procedure.

NOSE SURGERY

What Is Nose Surgery And What It Can Do

Nose surgery, known as rhinoplasty, is a very useful addition to facial cosmetic procedures. The nose changes with age and can also be corrected by surgery.

In some people, the tip of the nose may become bulbous. In others, it may begin to droop which results in a sharp angle between the nose and upper lip. The bridge of the nose may become more prominent and the nostrils may widen.

The aim of surgery is to restore the nose to its former shape or to restructure it to a more attractive shape. Noses that are very large or distorted are approached more radically. That is, more tissue is taken away and the nose shaped more extensively.

However, if the nose is normal in size or is only slightly larger than desirable, it is best to be conservative and aim for only subtle changes. It is far easier to remove tissue from a nose than to replace it.

How Nose Surgery Is Performed

Nose surgery can be either partial or complete.

Partial rhinoplasty is usually rapid and can be performed at the same time as a face-lift. It involves removal of some cartilage from the tip to reduce bulbousness or fullness. The cartilage removed can be placed under the nose deep into the upper lip. This acts as padding to elevate the nose tip.

Large nostrils can be reduced in size by cutting a small portion from their base.

Complete rhinoplasty involves more extensive restructuring of the cartilage and bone which forms its framework.

Both procedures can be done under local or general anesthesia.

Post-surgical dressings vary from doctor to doctor. They constitute a firm support to the nose to reduce movement during the healing period.

Most doctors will not use packs in the nose, especially when complete rhinoplasty is done. This may separate the bones and cause a deformity. Others may use small packs for a short time.

If any stitches are used on the outside of the nose, they are usually removed within four days and replaced with Steristrips. This holds the edges of the cut together until healing is complete.

Possible Side-Effects And Complications

It is best to visit a surgeon who has a lot of experience in rhinoplasty. Even though repair of an "overdone nose job" is possible by utilizing cartilage from the back of the ear, it is better to be conservative in changing the shape of the nose.

Possible complications after rhinoplasty include bleeding, swelling, bruising, asymmetry and infection.

A nose bleed is the most common of the complications, and usually occurs in the first two days, or between seven and ten days, following surgery. It is more common in older people whose tissues are more fragile and in those who resume physical activities, especially exercise, too soon after the operation. Cold packs to the back of the neck and head elevation stops most bleeding within ten to fifteen minutes. If bleeding continues, medical attention is required.

Swelling and bruising always occur in various degrees as with other surgical procedures. Elevating the head of the bed, cold compresses and reduced physical activity may help to limit the swelling. Some doctors use cortisone, injected intravenously during surgery, or tablets taken orally for a few days before and after surgery, to reduce the swelling. Excessive swelling can separate the surgically restructured bones and cartilage. This can lead to an undesirable cosmetic result. The most effective way of reducing post-surgical swelling and pain is the Diapulse.

Asymmetry may also occur. It may be corrected by further surgery. This should be delayed for a minimum of six months or until the tissues are completely healed.

Infection appears to be slightly more common following nasal surgery than other cosmetic surgical procedures. Many germs live in the nose. Even so, infection is generally rare.

Broken capillaries on the nose may occur in some patients particularly after several repeat procedures. These can be treated with the tuneable dye lasers (see Chapter 8).

FACIAL IMPLANTS
CHEEK AND CHIN AUGMENTATION

What Facial Implants Are And What They Can Do

Facial implants can be used to actually change certain facial structures to improve the overall appearance of the face. For example, they can create high cheek bones or build up the chin, if this is too small.

How Facial Implants Are Performed

Cheeks can be augmented in two ways. Either a permanent silastic implant of appropriate size and shape is inserted over the cheekbone through the inside of the mouth or through the lower eyelid.

Alternately, fat cells may be transplanted over the cheekbones. This procedure, however, is not permanent as the fat cells may not survive in their new location.

Chins can also be augmented in two ways. Either a permanent silastic implant is placed between the chin bone and muscle through a small cut inside the mouth or an incision under the chin.

Or, a portion of the chin bone is separated, moved forward and wired in place. This can be done through an incision in the mouth so there is no visible scarring.

Possible Side Effects And Complications

It may take some time to get accustomed to the new appearance. The augmentation may feel too prominent or not prominent enough. Both of these are easy to correct by further surgery. However, it is best to think about this carefully and make sure you have a good idea of what you are going to look like. The image computers, which are now available, may be an excellent way of seeing yourself with the implants before you go ahead with the surgery.

There may be the usual possible complications of bleeding, swelling, bruising and infection. Asymmetry is less likely than with other surgical procedures but may occur.

EAR SURGERY

What Is Ear Surgery And What It Can Do

Ear surgery is performed when the ears are facing forward too far instead of being located flat against the scalp.

Teasing can be a problem, especially for children and its psychological impact is a good reason for performing this procedure as early as 4 or 5 years of age.

How Ear Surgery Is Performed

Through a small incision behind the ear, a portion of the cartilage is either removed or folded onto itself and sewn together so that the ear is pulled back, flat, against the scalp.

A dressing is applied which is removed after several days or may be worn at night for comfort, for several weeks.

Possible Side-Effects And Complications

These are uncommon, but may include bleeding, asymmetry or infection. There will also be some discomfort until the healing is complete.

LIPOSUCTION

What Is Liposuction And What It Can Do

Liposuction is a relatively new procedure. It was first introduced in 1972 by a German plastic surgeon, Josef Schrudde.

Initially, there was great enthusiasm to remove enormous amounts of fat from obese people. This led to many serious complications, even death. The problems were widely publicized and gave liposuction a bad reputation.

Since then, liposuction has been more appropriately reserved for the correction of specific body contour problems. For example, for people who are not obese but have fat deposits, such as saddlebags on the thighs. These are difficult to lose by dieting and exercise alone.

Liposuction is not a weight-reducing procedure.

As a result of its more appropriate utilization, liposuction has become safe and effective. It can be performed in a doctor's office.

The best way to determine whether you would benefit from liposuction is to do the "pinch test." If you can comfortably pick up a substantial fold of skin which is separate from the underlying muscle, liposuction may be effective in removing the excess fat you feel between your fingers.

For the liposuction procedure, there has to be sufficient excess fat to fit the long thin liposuction rod between the muscle and skin and leave enough fat for an even surface.

Such fat collections occur most commonly in women on the side of the thighs (saddlebags), above the knees and sometimes around the ankles.

In these areas the overlying skin is fairly thick and the initial slackness after liposuction will tone up well. Generally, the younger patients' skin returns to normal.

In places where the skin is thin (beneath the chin, the upper arm, abdomen or inner thighs), it will become slack after fat removal and will tone more slowly. This is especially true in older people. In these cases, liposuction may be combined with surgical removal of the excess skin, which can leave visible scars that can be treated with lasers.

"Love handles" and buttocks present special problems.

Love handles are quite common in men, who otherwise are in great shape. Because the skin here is very thick, it is difficult to assess how much is fat and how much is skin. Even following removal of significant amounts of fat, it may take months for results to be seen. Thicker skin takes longer to tighten.

There are usually two reasons people are not happy with the shape of their buttocks: excess fat or lax muscles. Exercise or electro-muscle stimulation will help the latter problem, and liposuction will improve the first. But it is best not to expect too much fat to be removed from the buttocks. We need enough to remain as a cushion as well as for cosmetic appearance.

Cellulite May Or May Not Be Helped By Liposuction

Cellulite refers to the puckered appearance of skin in some areas of fat deposition such as the thighs. It occurs almost exclusively in women. It is thought to be caused by strands of tough tissue that run between skin and its undersurface, pulling the skin down between the collections of fatty deposits and thus creating dimples. The fat in these areas is no different to the fat in other parts of the body.

There are many treatments which claim to get rid of cellulite – creams, massage, exercise, even special diets. One that works with success is the loss of large amounts of fat through a healthy diet and exercise, which can be either active or passive. Liposuction may help in this regard, more by removing some of the fat, and less by breaking up some of the strands in between. The very hallmark of modern liposuction is the removal of fat without significant injury to other structures such as nerves, blood vessels and undersurface of skin, which causes scarring.

When enough fat is removed so that it no longer bulges between the strands of fibrous tissue, the appearance of the dimples may improve.

How Liposuction Is Performed

Liposuction can be performed under either local or general anesthesia, depending on the amount of fat to be removed. Liposuction is a fairly painful procedure. Extensive liposuction is best performed under general anesthesia. If pain can be eliminated, or if only small areas are being treated, there are advantages in doing it under local anesthesia. The patient can move or stand and fat can be removed more equally on both sides of the body. It is also easier to identify areas that may have been missed. Another advantage is that the patients see what has been taken out and give direction (within medically safe bounds), as to how much they wish to have removed.

On the day of surgery, you will be asked to shower at home with soap and water. Some doctors will give you antibiotics to take as a precaution to prevent infection.

If the procedure is performed following a numbing injection, a combination of anesthetic and sterile fluid is injected into the area and then deeply massaged to spread the fluid evenly.

When the area is adequately numb, a tiny cut is made in the skin. A long, thin, hollow tube (known as a cannula), which is connected to a pump, is introduced. When the pump is activated the fat is removed.

Alternatively, a syringe may be used in the same manner to withdraw the fat.

Afterwards a pressure dressing is applied. In addition to providing support, the pressure dressing also reduces the discomfort after the procedure. Especially in some of the more painful areas, such as the buttocks.

Possible Side-Effects And Complications

Since liposuction was first introduced, the incidence of all complications, especially the most serious ones, has been greatly reduced. Liposuction is now considered an effective and safe procedure.

A study of 10,000 cases of liposuction performed by dermatologists was recently published. The rate of minor complications such as irregularity, local bleeding and prolonged swelling, was reported to be 3 percent. More serious complications, including blood loss, infection, damage to underlying organs, and clots occurred in less than 0.5 percent of patients.

Bruising and discomfort can be expected during the first few weeks after surgery. Less commonly, discomfort may be experienced for several months. Avoiding strenuous exercise and wearing support garments will help to reduce the pain that is experienced.

The most common complication is irregularity of the skin surface, due to the removal of too much, or not enough fat. This can be corrected by massage, liposculpture, removing more fat, or putting some back if time alone does not solve the problem. Numbness or increased sensitivity may occur, but almost always goes away within five or six months.

Swelling can also be experienced. It is more common in sites such as the love handles and ankles. It can persist for some months and, in a few cases, up to a year.

Infections have been greatly reduced by careful attention to a sterile technique and preventative or early use of antibiotics.

LIPOSCULPTURE

What Is Liposculpture And How It is Used

Liposculpture was introduced to the United States a couple of years ago by an Italian physician, Dr. Marco Gasparotti. In this procedure, the fat just beneath the skin is removed, using less suction.

Liposculpture is claimed to have the following advantages: more fat may be removed, older patients with less skin elasticity can be treated, it can treat cellulite and correct irregularities caused by previous lipo-suction. It is also associated with the skin becoming tighter following the procedure. This effect is possibly due to fibrosis (scarring) which is stimulated to occur as high in the skin as the dermis by the trauma of repeat cannula insertions with little or no suction.

Possible Side-Effects And Complications

Liposculpture, like any new procedure, which lacks the comfort gained through time, is controversial. One of the main problems appears to be prolonged, purple "mottling" discoloration, unevenness and possible ulceration with consequent scarring which appears to occur when the skin is undermined with a hollow cannula without suc-tion, too close to the surface of skin.

Since the liposculpture technique is very new, it is not known whether the complication of purple mottling is permanent or resolves in time. It appears to take months or even years for this discoloration to fade, but so far does appear to be improving very slowly with time. The unevenness and scarring deeper in the tissues produce hardened, tender areas which appear to be more permanent. Laser treatment can correct only some of the most superficial scars.

The severity of the complications need to be considered very care-fully before deciding to go ahead with this procedure. It is crucial to select a physician who approaches this procedure with caution, a gen-tle, light touch, is not blindly over-optimistic or disregards the serious-ness of the possible complications, and above all, has a successful track-record in liposuction and liposculpture.

ABDOMINOPLASTY OR 'TUMMY TUCK'

What Is A 'Tummy Tuck' And What It Can Do

Abdominoplasty is the surgical removal of excess skin on the abdomen.

Pregnancies, fluctuations in weight, both weight loss and weight gain have the effect of causing skin over the abdomen to become per-manently stretched.

How The 'Tummy' Is 'Tucked'

This surgery is generally performed under general anesthesia. The skin is cut across the lower abdomen, just above the pubic area but below the bikini line.

Another incision is made around the belly button so that it can be freed from the surrounding skin which is then separated and pulled up over the lower ribs.

The abdominal muscles are tightened to improve the waist line. The skin is then lowered, a new opening, higher up is made for the belly button, and the skin is sutured together at the original incision line.

Afterward, a firm dressing is applied. A support garment is recommended for several months after surgery and strenuous activity should be avoided for at least a month.

Possible Side-Effects And Complications

There will be some bruising and soreness which can be relieved by keeping the hips bent to reduce strain on the abdomen for several days after surgery, by pain medication, and the Diapulse. The scar can become thickened and raised but can be treated with cortisone injections and lasers (see Chapter 8). Other complications include bleeding or uneven surface of the abdomen due to deeper scarring, which is beyond the reach of laser light. More severe complications (for example, involving the intestines) are rare.

BREAST SURGERY

BREAST AUGMENTATION, LIFT, REDUCTION AND RECONSTRUCTION

What They Are And What They Can Do

- Augmentation enlarges and shapes breasts when the breast tissue is small.

- Lift raises breast tissue back to its former position when it has dropped, due to age, gravity, pregnancy, breast feeding, and fluctuations in weight.

- Reduction reduces and reshapes large breasts by removing the excess skin and breast tissue. Excessively large breasts may cause problems including distorted posture, back ache, difficulty breathing and exercising, as well as skin irritation at the crease of the breast and unwelcome comments.

- Reconstruction rebuilds a breast after it is removed because of breast cancer. The latter procedure is called a mastectomy.

How Breast Surgery Is Performed

Breast Augmentation.

In this procedure, an implant is placed under the breast tissue or under the muscle, based on the surgeon's judgment and the build of the patient.

The incision for introduction of the implant is placed in one of the following sites:

1. In the armpit.
2. Around the areola (the darker skin around the nipple).
3. Underneath the breast, just where it touches the chest.

The different kinds of implants and their possible risks are outlined under silicone in this chapter.

Breast Lift and Reduction.

These procedures are similar. The incision lines are placed in an inverted "T", underneath where the breast meets the chest and in the center of the breast, from the chest to the areola.

The skin may also be cut around the areola, the breast tissue lifted to a higher, more youthful, former position, and any excess skin and breast tissue is removed.

If a lot of tissue needs to be removed, the areola and nipple may actually need to be completely detached before they are placed in the new position.

Breast Reconstruction.

This is a more complex, longer procedure.

If there is enough skin left after removal of the cancerous breast tissue, an implant can be used to reconstruct the breast. If there is not enough skin left, the remaining skin may be either 1) stretched by the use of a tissue expander, or 2) together with muscle and blood vessels to feed it, it may be taken from another area of the body, such as the back or abdomen. This is called a "flap."

1. A tissue expander is a device that looks like a balloon. It is placed under the muscle on the chest wall and over several weeks or months, gradually filled with fluid, thus stretching the overlying skin.

When enough stretch has occurred, an implant is placed under the muscle or the skin, at the discretion of the surgeon.

2. A flap consisting of skin, muscle and its blood supply is detached from its origin and moved as though through a tunnel to the breast area.

If the flap tissue is large enough to make up for the removed breast tissue, an implant may not be necessary. If not, an implant is placed under the flap.

The nipple and areola may need to be reconstructed at this time or at a later date.

Following all the different kinds of breast surgery, a dressing is applied or the patient dressed in a surgical bra which is worn for several days to a few weeks, depending on the extent of surgery. At that time, a softer bra should be worn for several weeks to months.

The stitches are removed within several days.

Breast augmentation is the least painful of these procedures with the patient returning to normal activities, except strenuous exercise within several days. Overhead lifting should also be avoided.

Breast reduction and reconstruction are more painful and have a longer recovery.

Possible Side-Effects And Complications

Apart from discomfort, there will be some bruising and swelling. The breasts will also feel more firm especially after an implant.

Some doctors recommend massage to soften the breasts.

The loss of sensitivity in the nipples will range from slight, temporary numbness to complete loss of sensation, depending on the degree of trauma to the areola and nipple areas.

Breast augmentation does not interfere with breast feeding; however, if the milk ducts leading to the nipple are severed as they can be during breast reduction, breast feeding will not be possible.

Also, if weight is put on after a breast lift or reduction, the breasts may enlarge and begin to drop again, requiring further surgery.

Scarring following breast lift, reduction and reconstruction may be quite prominent. Without laser treatment, the fading and flattening of scars is quite slow, taking considerably longer than six to twelve months. It can take as long as 5 to 10 years or even longer. Fortunately, these can be treated with specific laser techniques (see Chapter 8).

SCARS

Scars may occur whenever skin is cut. They may be red and raised, red and flat, or depressed. Or, they may be darker brown or whiter than the surrounding skin and atrophic — that is, thinner than the surrounding skin, having lost the normal skin texture — especially in areas that had sloughed or where the scars had stretched. All types of scars can now be treated by the use of specific laser techniques described in Chapter 8.

CHAPTER

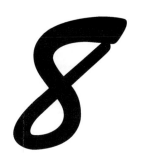

TREATING SKIN BLEMISHES

If we protect our skin from sunlight and inclement weather from early childhood, we will maintain the smooth, satiny, blemish-free complexion we were entrusted with at birth for a long time. Before tanned skin became the ideal, flawless skin at age forty was the norm.

Sun damage is responsible for virtually all acquired skin blemishes on the face and hands, including freckles, age spots, blotchy brown pigmentation, white spots where pigment was lost, and broken capillaries.

Some skin blemishes are present at birth, such as brown, black or red birthmarks, and moles. Those resulting from a multitude of skin diseases will not be discussed in this chapter.

CATEGORIES OF SKIN BLEMISHES

Skin blemishes can be divided into several categories:

1. Increased pigment: for example, freckles or age spots, melasma (pigmentation related to the pill or pregnancy), non-cancerous brown birthmarks, and pigment tattooed into skin.

2. Loss of pigment due to vitiligo, sun damage, or scarring.

3. Blood vessels on the face and neck: broken capillaries.

4. Blood vessels on the legs: spider and varicose veins

5. Scars: white, red, brown, depressed or raised, resulting from any cause.

Acquired Skin Blemishes

Freckles And Age Spots

Freckles are very common, especially in people who have red hair, and generally those with fair sun-damaged skin. These brown spots are made of collections of pigment cells in the top layers of skin. They are easily removed as long as they are freckles and not cancerous or pre-cancerous moles, in which case they have to be surgically removed and the diagnosis confirmed by a pathologist.

"Age" or "liver" spots are the larger brown spots found on the hands and sometimes on the forearms and face in later years. They too are the result of sun damage and have no relation to the liver.

Melasma

Melasma is pigmentation that develops in some people, typically on the cheeks and around the eyes. When the pigment is dark, it results in a "raccoon" look. It is aggravated by hormones, such as oral contraceptives, or during pregnancy, as well as, by sunlight. Melasma may improve after stopping the pill, delivery, or by avoiding sun exposure.

It is not only a very distressing problem to have, but is also very difficult to treat. Many methods have been tried over the years. No perfect treatment has been found as yet.

The problem with melasma is that treatments other than bleaching creams, Retin A and alphahydroxy acids (AHAs) can on occasion make the condition worse by either darkening the actual pigmentation or by making the normal surrounding skin lighter.

Non-Cancerous Brown Birthmarks

Non-cancerous brown discolorations of skin can be present at birth. They have different names depending on the color, site and structure.

The most common are moles, which vary in size from a pin-head to 6mm in diameter. If they are larger than this and have coarse hair growing out of them, they are not an ordinary mole. They are most likely a birthmark (if present from birth), called a giant hairy nevus, or a mole that may not be completely benign and require medical attention.

Cafe-au-lait spots can range in size from a five cent piece to covering large areas. They have the color of milk coffee, hence their name. Cafe-au-lait spots are quite common. However, they should be checked to verify they are definitely cafe-au-lait spots and not melanoma.

With a definite diagnosis as cafe-au-lait, the Q-switched Ruby or Q-switched YAG lasers can be used in place of surgical removal. It must be stressed that only benign lesions can be removed with lasers. Melanoma, suspicious moles and other skin cancers should be cut out and sent to a pathologist to confirm the diagnosis and make sure the lesions have been completely removed.

PIGMENT TATTOOED INTO SKIN

The most common unnatural pigment found in skin, is, of course, a decorative tattoo. As people grow older, it is common to decide they no longer want the tattoo.

In recent years, permanent eye make-up applied as a tattoo on the eyelids, eyebrows or lips has also been introduced. If not done carefully, it can leave permanent, unnatural marks that do not look attractive. Permanent eye make-up and tattoos can be removed with some lasers.

LOSS OF PIGMENT: VITILIGO AND SUN DAMAGE

Vitiligo is a skin condition in which the pigment cells die or stop producing pigment. This leaves white patches which may grow larger and eventually cover quite extensive areas.

The exact cause of vitiligo is unknown. It may be precipitated by many factors, like sunburn or stress, but can also appear without any cause.

It may not be particularly noticeable in people with very fair skin, but can pose a severe cosmetic problem in people with dark complexions. Laser treatment may help bring back pigment in some cases.

White spots due to sun damage may appear on the forearm and back after many years of sun exposure. These spots usually remain quite small, unlike vitiligo.

Broken Capillaries

Too many blood vessels, found too close to the surface of the skin, are commonly called "broken capillaries." They are dilated blood vessels medically known as telangiectasia.

They occur more commonly in people with fair skin who have either spent a great deal of time in the sun or who have suffered several sunburns especially in childhood. Broken capillaries are most numerous in sun-damaged areas, such as the cheeks, nose and neck. If sun damage is severe, they can cover the entire face, neck and arms.

Broken capillaries may be hereditary. This condition is called acne rosacea.

Regardless of the cause, all broken capillaries start as tiny pinpoint vessels. They first appear as a faint flush on the cheeks. The vessels continue to grow and can become quite prominent.

Heat, physical activity, embarrassment, alcohol and some spicy foods dilate these vessels, causing them to appear brighter red in color. They may all be associated with uncomfortably hot, painful, burning, stinging or itching sensations.

Sometimes small clusters of vessels can appear on other parts of the body. These are thin, spidery blood vessels, hence their name, "spider nevi" or spider angiomas. They sometimes appear in childhood and disappear without treatment. In adults, they may be caused by some medications, the pill or pregnancy, and can also be a sign of liver disease.

Spider And Varicose Veins

Spider veins are the streaks of spidery-looking vessels found on the legs. They occur almost exclusively in women. They first appear as thin red lines usually during the late twenties or after a pregnancy. They slowly increase in size and become large blue vessels. These large vessels may be associated with discomfort or aching, particularly after prolonged standing and in hot weather.

Varicose veins are the much larger, blue, bulging veins. Varicose veins may be aggravated by, or first appear during pregnancy and may improve after delivery of the baby.

The exact cause of varicose veins is obscure. They may be aggravated by hormones in women, increased pressure inside the abdomen which causes pooling of blood in leg veins, as occurs, for example, in pregnancy, and more rarely as a result of abnormal artery-vein connections. There may be a weakness of the valves in veins that connect the deep and superficial blood vessels. When the valves are faulty, blood flows backwards from the deep into the superficial veins, causing them to bulge. Normally, blood flows from the superficial blood vessels to the deep vessels and then back to the heart.

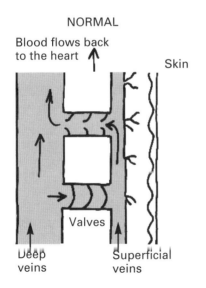
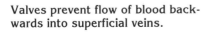
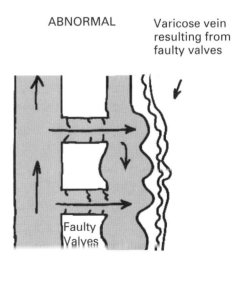

Valves prevent flow of blood backwards into superficial veins.

Faulty valves allow blood to flow backwards into superficial veins causing them to bulge resulting in varicose veins.

Varicose veins are generally hereditary. They may be associated with a deep ache and swelling of the legs, especially at the end of the day and in hot weather.

SCARS

Scars can be white, red or brown, raised or depressed. There are two types of raised scars: hypertrophic and keloid.

Hypertrophic Scars

Hypertrophic scars are red, raised, thickened scars that occur just in the line of deep injury such as a surgical cut especially in areas where the new wound is under tension. For example, on the back and abdomen. When the skin is strong enough, the body will slowly dissolve the thickened scar and leave a flat or depressed, white scar instead. It becomes white because the blood vessels that had grown in, to feed and help build the scar are absorbed when they are no longer needed and the scar lacks pigment cells.

The hypertrophic growth starts at about 2-3 months after surgery and reaches a maximum by 6-12 months. The thickened scar may then begin to regress of its own accord. However, the process of regression may be slow, in the range of 2-10 years or in rare instances even longer.

Keloid Scars

Keloids, on the other hand, are extremely thick, red, raised scars often associated with a severe itch and even pain, that grow beyond the margin of the original injury. They represent an over done healing process and can, for example, occur spontaneously, in response to acne, especially on the chest and back, a minor scratch and, of course, deep surgical or accidental injury.

Unlike hypertrophic scars, keloids are much thicker and do not go away with time. On the contrary, they may continue to grow larger, especially if surgical removal is attempted. For this reason, keloids are very difficult to treat. Surgical re-excision tends to make them come back larger than before. Radiation treatment and injection of cortisone may help. The carbon dioxide and argon lasers have been used successfully to treat these recalcitrant scars.

I have found alternating cortisone injections and laser treatment more helpful than either treatment alone.

Some people are more prone to developing keloids, for example Blacks and Asians. Keloids are also more common in younger people, on the chest, back and upper arms, following burns, and sometimes in association with acne. They are all notoriously difficult to treat.

POST-INFLAMMATORY PIGMENTATION

Some people have a tendency to develop darker brown pigmentation in scars. This can be temporary or permanent and can be triggered by minor injuries such as a scratch, superficial burn or sun exposure in the first few weeks following trauma or treatment to the skin. For example, following some chemical peels, dermabrasion or laser treatment. This is called post-inflammatory pigmentation and usually fades spontaneously within months of the injury. More rarely, it can be permanent and thus requires treatment for removal.

TREATMENT OF SKIN BLEMISHES

PROTECTION FROM THE SUN

Prevention Is Better Than Cure

Prevention is always better than cure. It is best to prevent sun-induced skin blemishes by avoiding excess sun exposure and always wearing sunscreen to protect the skin. This is absolutely crucial after some cosmetic procedures, such as a chemical peel, dermabrasion, or laser treatment. Even small amounts of sunlight (as little as five minutes of midday sun) can trigger pigment cells to produce more pigment (post-inflammatory pigmentation) in the immediate post-treatment period, that is, in the first two to four weeks.

If the original problem treated was pigmentation, sunlight can result in a recurrence or worsening of the problem. It is most important to remember that even minute amounts of sunlight, such as walking to and from your car to a nearby building, and certainly, driving without applying sunscreen in sunny *or cloudy* weather, is enough to stimulate pigment cells.

To make the situation even more difficult, it is not enough to protect just the affected area. This is because when tanning cells on any part of the body are exposed to the sun, they stimulate the remainder, those not directly exposed to the sun, to produce pigment. What this means is that if, after treatment to the face, the face and rest of the body are covered except the hands and feet which are exposed to the sun, the face may still develop darker discoloration. Applying a sunscreen with an SPF of at least 15 all over any skin exposed to the sun can prevent this problem. However, it is preferable to apply sunscreen and stay out of the sun.

BLEACHING AGENTS

What Bleaching Agents Are And How They Are Used

Bleaching agents contain various concentrations of a substance called hydroquinone, which makes up 1-7 percent of a cream or gel. Hydroquinone interferes with pigment production. After its use is discontinued, pigment cells resume their normal pigment production. Bleaching creams are often used to treat melasma, freckles and age spots.

After several weeks and sometimes several months of application, fading may be seen. However, this is only temporary (especially if the skin is exposed to the sun again after discontinuation of the cream) unless its use is combined with treatments that either remove the undesirable pigment and settle down or destroy some of the overactive pigment cells. Bleaching creams are very useful after chemical peels, dermabrasion and laser treatment. They reduce the initial "excitability" of the pigment cells.

Bleaching creams should not be used on a long-term basis. After many months of continuous use, they may turn the skin a slight yellow-orange color. Allergic reactions are also possible. If they occur, the bleaching cream should be discontinued.

FREEZING

What Freezing Is And How It Is Performed

Freezing is routinely used to remove small, superficial, benign brown spots and early skin cancers. It is not advisable for removing freckles that extend over a large area, such as the whole face or back, but can be used to remove individual freckles and age spots.

Carbon dioxide or nitrogen, in their liquid form, are very cold and are the agents used to freeze skin. They can be sprayed on or applied with a cotton-tipped applicator.

A burning or stinging sensation is experienced in the treated area for 5 to 20 minutes after application. Blisters may appear and are replaced by scabs that fall off within five to ten days.

Many doctors use this method frequently, and obtain excellent results without scarring.

In less experienced hands, especially in areas where skin is thin, like the back of the hands, the results may be less satisfactory. If the darker areas are frozen too deeply, a white spot may replace the brown spot. This, however, may be stimulated to repigment using laser light.

ELECTRODESSICATION

What Electrodessication Is And How It Is Used

Electrodessication uses heat to destroy individual broken capillaries or spider angiomas (not spider veins). It can also be used to destroy benign brown spots, but is employed less often for this purpose. It can be more painful and more difficult to apply evenly over a large, flat area, like a freckle or an age spot.

The instrument used to deliver heat is called a hyfrecator or cautery needle: a small piece of wire that resembles a ballpoint pen is heated electrically and applied to the spot on the skin to be destroyed. The healing time is similar to that following freezing.

CHEMICAL PEEL AND DERMABRASION

How They Are Used To Treat Blemishes

Chemical peels and dermabrasion can both be used to produce spectacular improvement of melasma on the face. They can also have little or no effect and on occasion, even make the pigmentation worse by darkening it or lightening the surrounding normal skin which accentuates the unchanged or darker color of the melasma pigmentation.

Unfortunately, testing a small area first will not necessarily predict the outcome when the whole area is treated later.

Dermabrasion used to treat acne scarring, may, incidentally, remove freckles. However, it is not suitable as the primary treatment of freckles, especially in young people.

Chemical peels can also be used to remove freckles and age spots, especially when these cover large areas like the face, back, arms and chest. However, if sunbathing is resumed after the peels, the freckles will eventually return.

Phenol produces a permanent loss of most, if not all, pigment cells. It is therefore suitable for those with fair skin who do not wish to tan afterwards. In those with suitable complexion, it can produce results unmatched by other less potent agents. It is suitable only for peeling the face. Chemical peels and dermabrasion are described in more detail in Chapter 7.

LASERS

What Lasers Are And How They Are Used To Treat Skin Blemishes And Improve Complexion Imperfections

Lasers are instruments that produce very intense, powerful beams of light. Different lasers produce different colors of light. Color and configuration of the laser light determine what effect the laser will have on the skin.

The past decade has seen an explosion in the number of medical lasers available, particularly in dermatology.

Lasers are a very useful advance in the treatment of some skin conditions such as tattoos, portwine and benign brown pigmented birthmarks, tuberous sclerosis, epidermal nevi, and now all manner of scars, sun-damaged skin and stretch marks for which there was previously no satisfactory treatment alternative. For other conditions such as age spots and freckles, where alternatives are available, the laser treatments may be faster and more reliable, and when lasers are used carefully and appropriately, removing the problem with a reduced risk of scarring.

Not all lasers are the same. There are many types. The optimal choice of lasers is determined by the type of condition to be treated and its depth in the skin.

The name of the laser refers to the name of the solid, liquid or gas that produces it. For example, argon laser light is produced by exciting argon gas; carbon dioxide laser light comes from carbon dioxide gas; the ruby laser light comes from the ruby crystal; while the light from the copper/gold vapor lasers is produced by vaporizing copper or gold metal.

The "dye" in a tunable dye laser, refers to a dye that is used inside the laser to produce a particular color of light. It doesn't go anywhere near the patient, as it does not leave the laser system, but works like fuel in a car. The light that comes out of a laser is pure light of a particular color.

Lasers should not be thought of as a magic cure for all skin conditions; nor should it be assumed that they are never able to cause scarring. **All lasers can result in scarring if high enough energies or long enough exposures are applied to cause a non-specific burn.** This is more difficult to do with the pulsed variety of lasers where the length of the laser exposure is limited by the laser type itself.

Nevertheless, even the pulsed variety of lasers can produce scars that are indistinguishable from a burn due to any cause. These burns are correctable by further *gentle* application often of the **same laser type as that which caused the scarring.** This shows clearly that **it is not the laser itself, but the method of application that is crucial in avoiding scarring.**

The continuous variety of lasers, including the copper vapor and KTP lasers are much more technique sensitive.

In the early 1980s, all the standard methods of applying laser light were associated with varying degrees of scarring ranging from 5% to 30% of patients treated.

I have developed and refined the methods of laser treatment which now make it possible to treat the conditions illustrated in this book. The techniques are very specific and tailored to each patient's skin. They are the result of fourteen years of experience in this field (eleven of which have been on a full-time basis), a personal refusal to accept the limitations of thinking that scars are permanent, and a desire to help people, especially those who have exhausted the conventional treatments and have nowhere else to turn.

However, good final results depend not only on the skill and experience of the operator, but also on the type of lesion, the patient's skin type, and, above all, how the patient's body responds to the treatment. The laser light does not actually remove the blemish. Rather, it stimulates our own body to remove it from inside the skin.

Thus, whether scarring can be removed completely depends largely on the individual patient's response.

Unique Properties Of Laser Light

1. **Selective Absorption.** Lasers are particularly suitable for the treatment of various skin blemishes due to their unique ability to produce concentrated beams of one color (monochromatic) light, which are more selectively absorbed by a particular pigmented tissue. However, the selectivity is not complete. Generally, about 90% of the laser light energy is absorbed by the targeted tissue, and 10% by the normal overlying or surrounding skin.

Which color of laser light is best absorbed is determined by the absorption spectra of different tissues. For example, hemoglobin, which gives blood its red color, best absorbs yellow and orange light, whereas melanin, the brown tanning pigment, best absorbs blue or green light. Thus by using different laser types, specific tissues can be destroyed while the overlying normal skin is spared from permanent scarring.

As melanin is a potential barrier to the incoming laser light, it is important to choose a wavelength that is better absorbed by hemoglobin than melanin when the desired end is to destroy superficial blood vessels. For example, the yellow or orange light from the argon dye or flashlamp-pumped pulsed dye lasers.

Conversely, when melanin-containing cells are the target, the wavelength or color of light chosen should be better absorbed by melanin than hemoglobin such as the red light of the Q-switched ruby laser or green light of the Q-switched YAG laser.

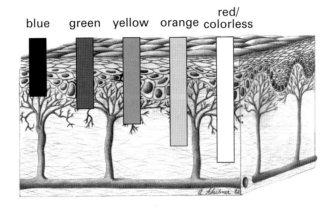

blue   green   yellow   orange   red/colorless

LIGHT COLOR (WAVELENGTH) AND SKIN PENETRATION

---

2. **Skin Penetration**. Another general property of light important in the selection of the appropriate wavelength is tissue penetration. The longer the wavelength, the deeper the tissue penetration. Thus, the red light from the Q-switched ruby laser or the colorless light from the Q-switched YAG laser is able to destroy dermal pigment more effectively than ultraviolet light even though the former is not as well absorbed by melanin, because the ultraviolet light is not able to reach pigment in the dermis.

3. **Configuration Of Laser Light**. Configuration of laser light refers to the shape of light coming out. For example, some lasers such as the argon, argon dye and carbon dioxide lasers produce continuous light. This can be interrupted by a mechanical shutter that "chops" light into shorter segments. These segments are sometimes referred to as pulses but they are not true pulsed light, they are quasi-pulsed light. True pulses of energy consist of a much larger burst of light.

Pulsed light sources such as the flashlamp-pumped pulsed dye laser, Q-switched ruby and Q-switched YAG lasers make light of very high energy which comes out in very short bursts or pulses. The total energy and duration of the pulse is set by the particular laser system. For example, the flashlamp-pumped pulsed dye laser produces pulses of 360 to 400 thousandths of a second while the Q-switched ruby laser produces pulses of 25-40 billionths of a second and the Q-switched YAG laser, pulses of 4-20 billionths of a second.

Pulsed light has an additional mechanical "shattering" effect which can be compared to that of an earthquake. The higher the energy and the shorter the pulse or burst of light, the greater the earthquake and the lesser the heating of the tissue targeted by the color of light. This fragmentation stimulates the immune system to remove the fragments of the unwanted tissue from inside the skin.

The copper and gold vapor lasers (the latter used only in photodynamic therapy — treatment of cancers with the help of a sensitizer substance) produce such rapid bursts of light that they appear continuous (quasi-continuous) to the naked eye and physiologically have the effects of continuous light on the skin, only more powerful.

The copper vapor laser produces its effect through heating rather than fragmenting because the "pulsed" light comes out continuously. Even when mechanically interrupted, it is not true pulsed light com-

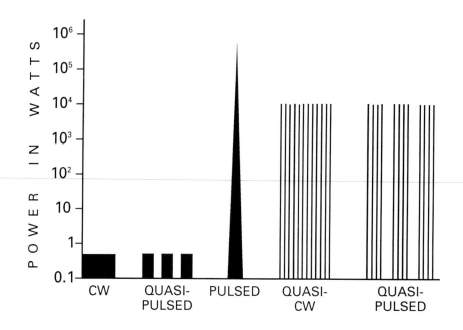

CONFIGURATION OF LASER LIGHT

pared to light from the flashlamp-pumped, Q-switched ruby and Q-switched YAG lasers. The copper vapor laser produces its effect by heating of target tissue in the skin which stimulates the body to remove the particular damaged tissue.

All lasers except the carbon dioxide laser, which destroys tissue directly by vaporizing it (turning it into smoke), produce their effects by damaging the segment in skin to be removed which stimulates the body to remove it.

Dangers

Patients often ask whether lasers are like X-rays. The answer is "No", they are nothing like X-rays. They consist of visible light of a particular color that has been shown not to produce or be associated with any malignant condition.

The light from the lasers under discussion here does not penetrate very deeply into the skin. Most penetrates only the top skin layers. Hence, its limitation in treating problems very deep in the skin, such as purple portwine stains or cavernous hemangiomas, unless the continuous light is held over one spot for very long periods of time using high energies, in which case it will produce non-specific burning of the entire tissue it is held over. This way, the light can be directed to go deeper into skin than it would otherwise penetrate based on its color alone. For example, the carbon dioxide laser is used as a cutting tool and can go through any human tissue if directed to do so.

The worst that could happen with the lasers discussed is that their inappropriate or indelicate use could result in burns and scarring. This, however, **can be corrected by further, very gentle application of laser light.**

The eyes of all participants are always protected as inadvertent exposure could result in damage to the unprotected eye.

How The Treatment Works

The laser beam passes through the normal overlying skin and the blood vessels or darker pigmented lesions selectively absorb the laser light thereby being sealed, exploded or coagulated (heated), depending on the laser type.

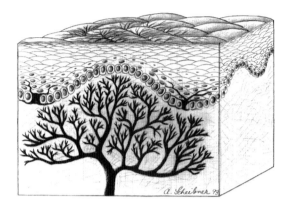

Excess broken capillaries in the upper dermis.

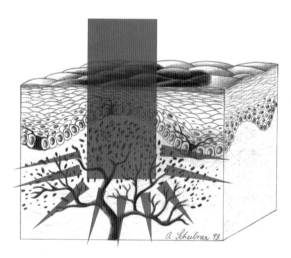

Pulse of light exploding small excess capillaries, which are not required for normal function of the skin.

The damaged specific tissue, such as the blood vessels, pigment cells or tattoo ink, is removed by the body by means of individual white blood cells, mostly within the first 5-6 weeks, but the area can continue to fade for 3-24 months after treatment. So, although, the effect of the laser is immediate, the final results are not seen for some time as improvement may continue to occur for many months. Maximal fading is seen at 3 to 4 months.

The difficulty and the skill necessary is to damage the blood vessels or any unwanted tissue under the skin without **excessive** burning of the overlying normal skin. Despite the most selective lasers (light exposed on the skin for extremely short periods of time), **some** heating of the overlying and surrounding skin does occur and may manifest itself as light scabbing and blistering and usually takes about 5-14 days to heal. The side benefit of this is that the skin may become tighter and smoother over the area treated as new collagen deposition is stimulated as illustrated in the photos on the next page.

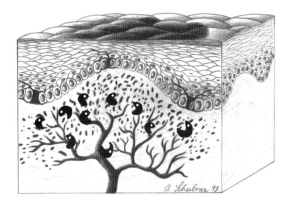

White blood cells removing fragments of the laser-treated unwanted tissue.

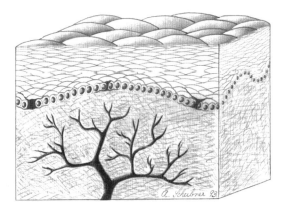

Normal blood vessels are restored.

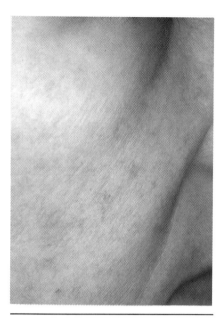

Result of chronic sun damage
before treatment.

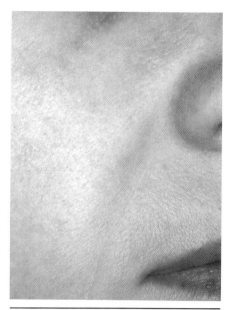

After laser treatment which resulted
in removal of broken capillaries
(less redness) and tightening of
skin due to new collagen formation
stimulated by the laser treatment.

What about repeat treatments?

Previously treated vascular areas that have responded only partially should be left to fade for at least 3-4 months, in some cases as long as 6 months, depending on the condition treated and the efficiency of the patient's re-absorption capacity. After this time, treatment can be repeated, if the blood vessels or pigmentation have not been completely removed.

The total number of treatments will depend on the number, size and depth of the vessels. The exact number of treatments cannot be predicted as this depends on many factors. The *average* number of treatments is as follows: Most broken capillaries take 1-2 treatments, larger ones 2-4. Those on the nose may need 2-6 and in rare cases even more treatments, as these are larger and generally tougher than elsewhere on the face. Age spots take 1-2 treatments and most scars, 2-4 repeat treatments, depending on the severity. Some of the more severe or extensive scars can require 8 or more repeat treatments.

Portwine birthmarks take the longest — a minimum of 4 treatments and could take as many as 20, or even more, repeat treatments. In fact, most birthmarks can be faded significantly and only a small percentage (10 to 20 percent) can be completely removed.

Does the treatment hurt?

The pulsed lasers, that is flashlamp-pumped dye, pigment lesion laser, Alexandrite, Q-switched ruby and Q-switched YAG, feel like the snapping of a rubber band. The majority of adults do not require an anesthetic of any kind. For extensive treatments, or those that require higher energies, local anesthetic injections or intramuscular Demerol and oral Valium may be used.

The continuous wave lasers, that is argon, argon dye, and quasi-continuous lasers; i.e., copper vapor and KTP feel like a hot pin touching the surface of the skin. Some adults do not require anesthetic for this treatment. Most do. Topical lidocaine cream (made by a pharmacist with a doctor's prescription) is generally sufficient to numb the surface of the skin to remove or at least reduce the burning sensation.

After the first 2-3 minutes of continuous laser treatment, the skin being treated becomes less sensitive so that the "pin-prick" is felt only when the laser light is moved to a new, untreated area.

The copper vapor application tends to feel more uncomfortable than the argon dye and pulsed dye lasers.

Children are treated under sedation or general anesthesia administered by an anesthesiologist or anesthetist.

In Summary

Of the most commonly used, there are six types of lasers to treat skin blemishes:

1. The argon dye laser produces yellow or orange light best absorbed by hemoglobin and is used for the medium to large-sized vessels such as those in purple portwine stains and broken capillaries on the nose.

The argon laser produces blue and green light. It is used to treat brown discoloration as well as to smooth texture of the skin. For example, surgical, accidental and acne scarring and wrinkles around the lips. Wrinkles caused by movement such as smiling are not suitable as the repetitive motion, which caused them in the first place, is likely to bring them back quickly. Collagen injections are the best treatment for such wrinkles.

2. The carbon dioxide laser produces colorless light that is best absorbed by water. Since most of the body tissues are composed of 70% water, all will absorb this laser light. At high energies and a small spot of laser light, the tissue will be instantly vaporized or "cut." The carbon dioxide laser is used as a cutting instrument in surgery or to destroy undesirable tissue such as warts and skin tags.

3. The flashlamp-pumped pulsed dye laser produces pulses of yellow or yellow-orange light that heat and rupture the smallest vessels (less than one-tenth of a millimeter in diameter) such as those in pink and red portwine stains and most broken capillaries.

4. The pigment lesion laser produces pulses of green light that are best absorbed by superficial pigment such as age spots. This laser is not suitable for the treatment of pigment deeper in the skin.

5. The Q-switched ruby and Q-switched YAG lasers are used to treat tattoos and brown skin discoloration, such as freckles, liver spots and some brown birthmarks, especially those in which the pigment is deep in the skin.

6. The copper vapor and copper bromide lasers are similar to the argon dye laser, but produce more intense light, as it comes out in rapid pulses with high energy peaks. These are so frequent that the light appears continuous. It is not suitable for people with fine skin, as this is more easily burnt and, therefore more easily scarred.

The KTP laser produces green light that also comes out in pulses so fast they appear continuous to the naked eye. Its applications are similar to the copper vapor and copper bromide lasers.

The gold vapor laser produces rapid pulses of red light that also appear to be continuous to the naked eye. It is used in photodynamic therapy for the treatment of inoperable cancer.

What can be treated?

- Excess or unwanted blood vessels.

- Portwine stains.

- Broken capillaries on the face.

- The smallest red vessels on the legs (larger ones are best injected as they respond better to injections with sclerosing solution).

- Spider angiomas - the small "spidery" vessels mostly on the face, but which can occur on any body site.

- Cherry angiomas - the more distinct, rounded and raised red spots on any body site.

- Sun damaged skin on the face and neck (Poikiloderma of Civatte).

- Acne rosacea - a hereditary condition of developing broken capillaries on the face earlier in life than would be expected as a result of sun damage alone.

- Rare conditions such as Rothmund-Thompson syndrome where excess broken capillaries are very close to the surface of the skin.

These conditions are described as superficial blood vessel malformations and are made up of a network of blood vessels which, because of their closeness to the skin surface, give the skin a red or blood color. Many methods have been tried to correct these lesions (such as excision, cauterization, etc.); however, none, other than **appropriately** used lasers, have given consistently satisfying, lasting and scar-free results.

Scars

- Hypertrophic.
- Keloid.
- Accidental due to windshield injuries, dog bite, etc.
- Surgical – any time skin is cut deeply beyond the regenerative basal layer at the dermo-epidermal junction, it may heal with a permanent scar.
- Acne.
- Chicken pox.

- Burns.

- White scars from any cause including stretch marks.

- Scars resulting from complications of collagen and silicone injections.

Pigment Cell Lesions

- Liver spots (have nothing to do with the liver except that their color, shape and often large size resemble the liver in appearance).

- Freckles.

- Post-inflammatory pigmentation, i.e. pigmentation that may develop following any procedure such as a peel, laser treatment, sclerotherapy or trauma such as burns, or accidental injury.

- Cafe au lait spots, "milk coffee" patches present at birth.

- A number of more rare brown or black birthmarks such as Becker's nevus, Nevus of Ota and Ita (more common in people of Asian descent).

Only benign pigmentation is suitable for treatment. Pigmented moles are best biopsied or excised to determine the exact diagnosis and to exclude the possibility of melanoma. Lesions such as giant hairy nevi which have a risk of developing a malignancy are best excised if small enough. However, with larger lesions, especially very extensive lesions on the face, the psychological trauma of such a severe disfigurement can outweigh the small risk of a potential malignancy. The most superficial problems such as liver spots and freckles can be treated with lasers, freezing with liquid nitrogen, or a light peel.

Tattoos

The ruby laser was the first laser ever built in 1960. It was also the first laser used in dermatology. Its initial use with very high powers resulted in so much scarring that it was abandoned until Professor Reid in Glasgow, Scotland began using this laser with an adaption — the Q-switch. This enabled tremendously high laser energies to be delivered in an extraordinarily short period of time: 40 billionths of a second.

This, together with low energies, prevented any burn to the normal overlying skin but fragmented the tattoo ink. After 10 years of producing consistently excellent results in removing tattoos, the Scottish group were still not taken seriously.

When I first heard about these treatments in 1988, I visited Glasgow and confirmed the unsurpassed excellence of the results. Prior to this, other lasers had been used to burn out the pigment and the normal overlying skin resulting in moderate to severe scarring ranging froming 5 to 30 percent, while minor scarring consisting of a change in skin color or texture almost always occurred. In general, this was still less than the alternatives, such as excision, skin graft or deep dermabrasion.

I was truly inspired by the results, and was instrumental in the development of a viable Q-switched ruby laser system where previously only the scientific laser system was available. Work at Harvard Medical School by Rox Anderson, M.D. resulted in FDA approval by the end of 1989. The Q-switched ruby laser best removes blue and black ink. It does little for colored tattoos, especially "ignoring" the yellow color.

Since then, Dr. Rox Anderson and his group have investigated and found the Q-switched YAG laser to be even better in the removal of tattoos. The light from this laser is even more powerful, coming out in pulses of 4-20 billionths of a second. It is better able to remove color, including red* and yellow ink.

I have found the application of a light fruit acid pool, called Jessner's solution, to the treated area immediately after the laser treatment to accelerate removal of the tattoos. This includes red, green and yellow pigments which without this additional step normally take many repeat treatments: ten or more not being unusual.

Also, the skin in dark or tanned individuals is less transiently hypopigmented (whiter than usual) following the Q-switched YAG laser treatment. The Q-switched ruby laser is still very useful in the treatment of pigmented lesions where the pigment is deep in the skin.

Permanent Make-Up

This requires a word of caution. Although it is possible to remove

---

* Removal of red ink can cause serious allergic reactions in the immediate post-treatment period.

make-up tattooed into the skin for the purpose of being permanent, the process involved requires repeat treatments and carries the risk of the flesh-colored pigments containing iron oxide turning instantly black, grey or green upon contact with laser light from the Q-switched YAG or ruby lasers.

This darker pigment can be removed with further laser treatments. The removal process can be accelerated by the application of a light fruit acid peel immediately after each laser treatment and for several days afterward. The process of removal is slow, the treatments being spaced about 2 to 6 weeks apart to allow the body enough time to reabsorb the unwanted pigment.

It is therefore best to consider very carefully whether to have permanent make-up, to choose the shape and color with precision, and ascertain the experience and skill of the professional doing the procedure (see Chapter 9).

Other Benign Skin Growths

- Skin tags.

- Epidermal or warty nevi (specific, rare birthmark not the usual mole or nevus).

- Non-pigmented, compound nevi.

- Skin lesions of tuberous sclerosis - benign, red, raised rounded growths on the face similar in nature but much smaller than that of the "Elephant Man."

Pores

The large size of pores may be partly the result of the skin becoming lax, as normally occurs in time. This results in shadows which make the pores appear larger as illustrated in Chapter 5. The solution is to tighten the skin between the pores.

Lasers can be used to tighten skin between pores by stimulating new collagen formation which results in the skin becoming tighter and, therefore, smoother. Light and medium peels will have a similar effect.

Pores can also appear larger when they fill up with sebaceous secretions. When these are not extracted fast enough, they can distend the pore. In addition, the top portions of this material can oxidize, which results in dark grey and eventually black discoloration. Regular exfoliation helps to remove this sebaceous material and prevents excess build up as described in Chapter 5.

What Happens After Treatment?

Argon, Argon Dye, Copper Vapor, Q-Switched Ruby, and Q-Switched YAG Lasers

24 Hours: If the skin is very fine and delicate, there may be some blistering; this usually resolves within 24-48 hours. As the blisters collapse, they are replaced by very fine, superficial scabbing which resembles "cat-scratch" marks.

1-7 Days: If blistering has occurred, this will peel in a similar way to skin that has been sunburnt. However, it is important not to force any peeling prematurely which may cause depressions in the skin. If these do not resolve in time, they may be removed with further laser treatment.

The treated areas should be kept clean by washing with lukewarm water once or twice a day. It is advisable not to use harsh soaps, as these may dry the skin too much. A moisturizer such as vitamin E oil or antibiotic ointment can be applied 2-4 times a day during the first 1-2 weeks following treatment. It is preferable that the skin be kept moist and not too dry as this may lead to cracking and bleeding in the immediate post-operative period.

7-14 Days: The face generally is completely healed — that is, there is no crusting. Slight redness may be present for an additional two weeks or so. It may take an additional 6-12 weeks to see the final result of the one treatment, as remnants of the targeted unwanted tissue continue to be cleared away and new collagen is stimulated to form.

1-3 Months: The arms, trunk and legs generally take longer to heal. The targeted vessels begin to break down and become burgundy red to rusty brown in color and may take from one to several months to be completely reabsorbed. In some instances, it may take 6-12 months to reabsorb completely. This is one reason why lasers are not the best treatment for spider veins on the legs.

Flashlamp-Pumped Pulsed Dye And Pigmented Lesion Lasers

Immediately upon application of a 3mm to 5mm spot, the area turns a purple color. It continues to darken over the next 24 to 48 hours, reaching the deep purple/black color of eggplant. After this time, the purple begins to fade rapidly to lighter purple, rusty brown, then pink, and is completely absorbed in 2 to 4 weeks without added therapy to accelerate healing. Treatment close to eyes or over extensive areas can cause moderate to severe swelling for 2 to 5 days.

With the help of Diapulse therapy immediately after, and then 15 to 30 minutes a day for several days, the healing time is reduced by half, approximately 1 to 2 weeks of purple, rusty brown and pink discoloration. However, the exact healing time varies from patient to patient.

Final Results

At the end of this time, the skin looks the same as it did before treatment. That is, unchanged or evenly slightly discolored with a "pink haze" which may last an additional two to four weeks. The maximum improvement is not seen for another 3 to 4 months and further improvement continues for two years or even longer.

COSMETIC TREATMENTS FOR HANDS

Possible Options

Treatments available for hands deserve special mention.

Rejuvenation of the skin on the hands has long been of concern to women, particularly when the rejuvenated face does not match the hands.

Hands are, in general, more difficult to treat because the skin is thin, easily damaged and more prone to scarring.

The two cosmetic procedures beneficial for hands are the removal of age spots and the replacement of the fat that has been lost from the back of the hands. The loss of fat makes the tendons and veins visible.

Microlipoinjection, described in the previous chapter can replace the lost fat. A number of treatments are available for age spots such as bleaching, freezing, chemical peels and laser treatments.

The laser treatments are the most specific and if performed correctly, carry the least risk of scarring. Freezing is the most likely to leave white spots instead of the dark brown age spots. These white spots can be treated either with specific laser techniques as described above or repigmented with dermapigmentation (see Chapter 9).

More than any other part of our body, the hands are exposed to many detrimental environmental stresses: frequent use of soap and water; contact with various chemicals (household and industrial); extremes of temperature; and probably more sun exposure than the face.

It is best to protect the hands by avoiding excessive contact with soap and water, wearing protective cotton gloves under rubber gloves when washing, or handling chemicals, and applying protective creams containing sunscreens.

LASER FACE-LIFTS

In the last few years, a number of articles have appeared promoting the advantages of using laser light, produced by the carbon dioxide laser, as a cutting tool in various cosmetic procedures such as eyelid reduction (blepharoplasty) or face lifts.

How The Carbon Dioxide Laser Is Used

The light produced by the carbon dioxide laser is best absorbed by water. Since most body tissues are composed of 70 percent water, a very small spot of this type of laser light will have the effect of "cutting" tissue by vaporizing it (turning it into smoke) in a fine-line, at the point of contact. Thus, it works like a *scalpel of light.*

Some surgeons believe it has definite advantages over the conventional scalpel — others disagree. The list of advantages include:

- Less bleeding as the heat from the light seals blood vessels as it cuts through tissue.

- This allows the surgeon to have a clearer view of the area and therefore work more effectively.

- It also reduces bruising so that the patient is presentable sooner.

Possible Complications And Precautions

- Some surgeons believe that the laser-cut edges which are charred need to be cut away with a scalpel later to prevent scarring. They also believe that bleeding and bruising are related to the patient's tendency to easy bruising and the surgeon's skill and experience and not the instrument he uses.

- More risk of scarring and infection if the charred edges are not removed.

- The laser procedure takes longer to perform.

- There is a risk of accidental burn to the skin or the eyes which in the worst scenario could cause blindness, if the carbon dioxide laser is used by a surgeon who is not experienced in its use.

- It is more expensive.

SCLEROTHERAPY

The Injection Of Varicose Veins And Spider Veins

Sclerotherapy is the injection of unwanted veins. A sclerosing solution is injected that damages the lining of the vessel wall. The damaged vessel is sealed and removed by the body.

Various sclerosing fluids are used for this purpose. The most common is concentrated salt solution, which is the most "natural" and does not cause allergic reactions. Stronger agents may be required to treat varicose veins.

The injection of varicose veins remains controversial. Varicose veins have traditionally been treated by vascular surgeons, with a surgical procedure called ligation and stripping. The rationale for this operation, and the main objection to sclerotherapy, is that the faulty perforators, blood vessels that bridge the deep and superficial veins in more than 200 locations on the leg, need to be closed off to cure varicose veins.

Because pressure in the deep venous system is relatively high, it is claimed to be difficult to effectively close perforators and eliminate varicose veins with injections alone. Tying these vessels, that is, ligating them, is supposed to be more full-proof.

In practice, this is not always the case, as it is not possible or desirable to tie off all the perforators. Neither injections nor surgery have been found to cure all varicose veins. Two to three years after injections and five to six years after surgery, a certain percentage of varicose veins come back and require further treatment.

The advantage of sclerotherapy is that if done correctly, it does not leave surgical scars. It can also be done as an outpatient procedure without anesthesia and with little or no discomfort.

The procedure that is gaining acceptance in the medical profession is a combination of surgery and sclerotherapy. If there are faulty (incompetent) perforators, they are first tied through a small incision in the overlying skin. The remaining varicose veins are then injected rather than removed (stripped) surgically. More women now know about the alternatives to surgery and can make their own decisions about treatment.

How Sclerotherapy Is Performed And What You Can Expect

Sclerotherapy to treat either spider or varicose veins is very similar. Solution is injected using small needles to eliminate discomfort. The patient usually sits or reclines.

Some sclerosants sting while being injected, others are painless. Concentrated salt solution is the most commonly used. It is mixed with a small amount of novocaine which virtually eliminates any stinging sensation. Although, the most "natural," salt solution is also the most difficult to use as it needs to be injected with **precision**. If a large amount is injected outside the vein, an ulcer can develop. This is avoidable by careful, steady injection. Even if a small amount were injected outside the vein, it can be diluted by injection of some novocaine, which prevents any possible ulcers from developing.

It is best to avoid strenuous exercise, such as jogging or aerobics for the first week. Gentle exercise such as walking and swimming are recommended immediately. Compression stockings worn for several days afterwards will help to close the veins.

Apart from the possible initial discomfort, little is felt afterwards, except when larger veins respond very quickly, in which case there may be some tenderness directly over the involved vein. However, this is only mild and responds to aspirin.

Severe or even mild pain in the calf, redness, swelling and heat are not normal and may indicate a deep vein clot which requires immediate medical attention. This is a very rare complication of deep varicose vein and perforator injections.

It takes two to six weeks for the results of treatment of spider veins to become apparent and up to two to six months for varicose veins. It may take even longer than this for treated veins to clear, if a laser is used to treat the smallest spider veins.

Possible Complications And Precautions

Because the sclerosant can damage anything it has contact with, there is a risk of ulceration developing at the injection site. Solution can leak through the needle track or be accidentally injected outside the vein. Unless particularly large, most ulcers caused by sclerotherapy will heal without scarring. If scars do occur, they can be treated with specific laser techniques.

Certain sclerosants and sometimes injection of larger vessels may occasionally result in dark brown pigmentation developing over the vessel. Some discoloration is normal and is due to the products of hemoglobin breakdown, which are brown. Hemoglobin is the red pigment in blood. In the majority of people, the brown color is eventually reabsorbed, although it may sometimes take as long as two years. This pigmentation can also be removed faster than with time alone, with certain laser techniques or gentle peeling agents.

Another possible complication is a matt of tiny vessels which may sometimes appear at the site of the injection. Fortunately, most matts will go away without treatment. If they do not, the vessels may be removed with further injections of tiny amounts of solution or sometimes lasers may be used to remove them.

ACCELERATING THE HEALING PROCESS

DIAPULSE TECHNOLOGY

What Diapulse Is And How It Is Used

The Diapulse machine was first developed by Abraham Ginsberg, M.D., in 1941, to eliminate the dangers of heat and introduce pulsed high frequency electromagnetic energy, in treatment of edema and pain. It has been in international clinical use for 35 years, and has extensive documentation by research studies performed in leading universities and hospitals, published in peer review medical journals.

Diapulse has been proved to be completely safe. The recent press reports regarding dangers of electromagnetic waves refer to low frequency, as generated by power lines, TV, and so on, with entirely different parameters than Diapulse.

In fact, the Diapulse parameters cannot be compared with any other device, such as ultrasound or electrical stimulation.

Diapulse treatment is painless. It is administered by placing the area to be treated in contact with the drum of the unit, for 15 to 30 minutes for the prescribed course of treatment depending on the extent and nature of the wound, as well as the general condition of the patient. The course could range from one to several days, or weeks.

Treatment can be applied effectively through surgical dressings or clothing, and may be indicated before surgery as well as after.

Treatment dramatically reduces post-operative bruising, incidence of hematoma formations (under the skin bleeding), swelling and pain. Suture time is reduced by several days; scarring is minimized by the faster healing, and pain medication is often eliminated entirely.

A simple explanation of Diapulse technology: living cells have electrical and chemical balance which is disturbed due to damage such as surgery or any procedure or accidental injury. Sodium and water move into the cells causing swelling (edema). Nature's process slowly removes the sodium and water over a period of 4 to 6 days in healthy tissue, and longer than this if the circulation or healing are impaired. Healing cannot occur until the edema is reduced. Diapulse rapidly restores the normal tissue equilibrium, and edema frequently is prevented from forming – or is quickly reduced.

Research demonstrates that Diapulse:

- Increases blood flow to the involved area, thereby increasing oxygenation of tissue.

- Accelerates collagen deposition.

- Accelerates removal of any laser-treated tissue.

- Reduces healing time by as much as 50% following surgery, laser treatment or peels.

Applications

Published research indicates the value of Diapulse technology in conditions with evidence of edema and pain due to:

- Post-operative swelling and pain.

- Acute injuries to bones.

- Recalcitrant wounds such as pressure sores.

Contraindications And Precautions

As with all electrical devices, Diapulse should not be used on patients with electronic pacemakers, with metal implants in the area of application, patients who are skeletally immature, or during pregnancy.

C H A P T E R

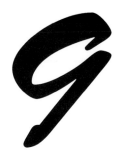

DERMAPIGMENTATION OR COSMETIC TATTOOING*

The concept of permanent make-up (cosmetic facial tattooing) has been in existence for hundreds of years. More recently, the procedure has become very popular in the Orient, especially countries such as Korea, Taiwan and Japan.

The concept of permanent make-up is relatively new in America and appears to be gaining popularity. *When performed well by an experienced and skillful operator,* the advantages are readily apparent, especially for women who have difficulty putting on or keeping on their make-up. For example, arthritis sufferers, those with make-up allergies or poor vision, and swimmers or other athletes who are concerned about make-up washing off or running. Permanent make-up is also useful for women who wear contact lenses. The most popular procedure appears to be the eyeliner. However, permanent eyebrows, lip line and full lip color (replacing lipstick) are now fairly common procedures.

---

*Information on dermapigmentation provided courtesy of the American Institute of Permanent Color Technology.

MACRO-THEORY DERMAGRAPHICS

What Macro-Theory Dermagraphics Is And How It Is Used

This technique involves the implantation of pure iron oxide pigment into the dermis, or deeper layer of the skin. With topical anesthesia, it is a relatively painless, non-surgical procedure which can be performed on an out-patient basis.

The concept of Macro-Theory Dermagraphics is similar to standard tattooing. However, the technique of application is more delicate, being closer to the techniques of electrolysis, which are very precise and require extensive training. Macro-Theory involves a delicate, controlled method of applying subtle micro-insertions of pigment into the skin. The idea is to form a natural shadow of color on the skin, achieving a gentle *natural* look (as opposed to the harshness of a standard or *drawn* tattoo line).

Pigment is placed into the dermis, and as the settling and healing process takes place over the following weeks, the epidermis covers the pigment. This produces a *fuzzy* effect that looks natural. The swelling is usually minimal, and most women are able to return to work the following day.

The sensation has been described as similar to plucking an eyebrow or experiencing a pin-pricking sensation across the skin. A topical anesthetic may also be applied.

How This Procedure Is Performed

Unlike a standard tattoo which is basically drawn on in a matter of minutes, this procedure takes approximately an hour, and is designed to be applied in stages. Due to the subtlety of the implants, you receive a basic shape and color on the first "saturation" visit. You then return for a "focus" visit to add the fine detail to the eyebrow or liner that has been applied.

Pigment colors are best selected to imitate the multitude of natural colors one sees in eyebrows and eyelashes, as well as, skin tones. Soft pinks and corals can be applied to the lips to enhance their shape and provide definition.

The pigment is applied with a sterilized instrument resembling a large marking pen. When gripped like a pencil, the machine can be used to insert pigment in small areas. Either one, or a cluster of micro-needles are used to introduce the pigment into the skin.

A series of two or three more subtle treatments enables a natural progression of color guided by you, as you observe the applications to adjust and identify the precise shape, color and contrast you want. The visual effect is "soft focus," creating a natural appearance.

This procedure allows a step-by-step construction of the desired feature enhancement to achieve exactly what you want.

The advantage of this procedure is that you are directly involved in all decision-making. This enables you to actually look in a mirror and guide the technician. This is very important as it may take you some time to adjust to your new appearance. If the added pigmentation is very different to your usual make-up or applied in one large step, you may panic and decide you don't like your new appearance after the pigment has already been implanted.

Immediately after the treatment, the skin can be slightly swollen. Ice or the Diapulse can be used to reduce any swelling. The treated area usually appears normal within a few hours after the procedure.

A Typical Treatment Schedule

At the initial visit, you need to evaluate your present make-up and decide how you want to look. Consider color and shape as being the two most important factors.

Consultation: should take place five to seven days prior to the actual treatment to discuss the desired procedure, complete patient history, and have an allergy test. If the procedure is eyebrows, all **unwanted** hair is first removed in the treated area. Bring all your cosmetics to demonstrate the desired effects. Photos may be taken.

First Saturation Visit: One hour appointment. The color reaction to the pigment is tested. "Before" photos are taken without makeup. The Macro-Theory procedure is performed. Note: It is not realistic for you to look at a procedure immediately upon the conclusion of an application, to determine what it will eventually look like (ten days later). No soap, no sun, and no makeup for five days following the procedure. No driving for 8 to 10 hours following an eyeliner procedure due to possible swelling.

Second Saturation Visit: Up to one hour appointment, two weeks after the first saturation visit. The purpose is to adjust the application method (probe angle and depth), as well as pigment color as needed for accurate and thorough saturation (based on observation of results from first saturation visit). The same restrictions apply as with the first saturation visit. Photos may be taken.

Third Saturation Visit: If necessary. Same as second visit.

First Focus: You guide the Derma-Tech, using a mirror, to achieve exact details of both shape and color (for example: definition of borders and adjustment of color).

Second Focus: If necessary. Same as first focus.

Medical Applications

The applications of this procedure within the realm of medicine are numerous. Conditions such as alopecia (hair loss), where patients receive the appearance of eyebrows and eyelashes, and the eyeliner technique for patients whose physical limitations make applying eyeliner difficult, are the most common procedures prescribed.

Thousands of women who have difficulty in applying eye make-up or are allergic to the ingredients in certain cosmetic preparations can receive the benefits of permanent eye make-up. Women with arthritis or neurologic problems, who have painful or unsteady movement of the hands, who cannot see without corrected vision when applying make-up, and women with oily skin or tearing eyes are typical eyeliner candidates.

In the past few years, corrective camouflaging has emerged as a useful service to dermatologists and plastic surgeons when they can no longer medically improve a patient's appearance. For example, vitiligo and white scars when laser treatment is not available.

Dermapigmentation can help correct features, such as a cleft lip, and with caution even improve the appearance of the basic facial shape, in some select cases.

It has also been applied to cover stretch marks. Burn survivors and patients suffering from scarring after basal cell carcinoma removal can benefit from the camouflaging effect of the procedure.

Areola re-pigmentation, often provided by plastic surgeons, has proved an effective technique to recreate the natural appearance of the areola and nipple after breast reconstructive surgery. The procedure has also been used to fill the spaces between transplanted hair grafts to improve the cosmetic result of hair transplant procedures.

Commonly Asked Questions

Q: Can I wear additional makeup over my permanent color?

A: Yes. Macro-Theory applications generally provide a subtle look for natural feature enhancement. You still may choose to apply "night" makeup for a more glamorous appearance.

Q: Is dermapigmentation permanent?

A: All pigments will eventually fade, some after eight to ten years, others earlier or later so that re-treatment may be required.

Q: Does it hurt?

A: Except around the eyes, the treatment is quite tolerable. Eyelids can be treated with a topical anesthetic before treatment.

Q: What if I am allergic to the pigment?

A: A sensitivity test is performed prior to all procedures. Generally, the pigment is applied to a small "patch" area behind the ear. A waiting period of about two weeks allows the Derma-Tech to observe any reaction.

Q: Can I get an infection?

A: Infection is possible with any procedure which breaks the skin. Check the references and credentials of your Derma-Tech so that you may feel confident about your procedures. The American Institute of Permanent Color Technology in Irvine, California provides listings of qualified Derma-Techs certified in Macro-Theory Dermagraphics (see Bibliography).

Possible Complications and Precautions

Warnings about crooked lines or running, permanent eyeliner have been widely published. Removal is possible and can be done using either the Q-switched YAG or the Q-switched Ruby lasers. However, both will initially discolor flesh-colored iron oxide pigments black, grey or green. These then require repeat treatments to remove as do other black, grey or green tattoos. It is therefore best to avoid removal by careful selection of the technician and careful consideration of the shape of the desired permanent make-up. Choose the person who is going to treat you very carefully; remember, you are having **permanent** eyeliner or eyebrows applied.

P H O T O S E C T I O N

The following "before" and "after" photographs of scar and sun damage treatment are the result of techniques I have developed which are patent-registered.

At present these techniques are available at practices in Beverly Hills, Ojai, and Palm Springs, California, and Sydney, Australia.

I have to date treated over 10,000 scars and continue to treat several hundred a week.

Stretch marks before laser treatment.

After one laser treatment using these specific techniques.

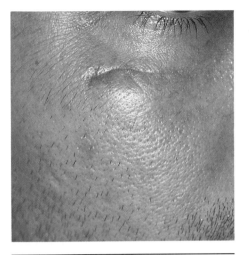

Cheek scar before laser treatment.

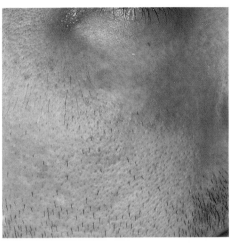

After three repeat laser treatments.

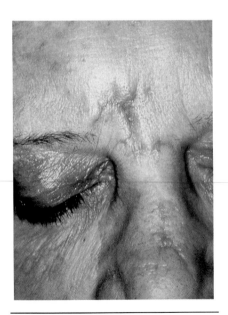

Forehead scar before laser treatment.

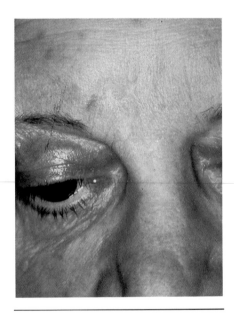

After four laser treatments.

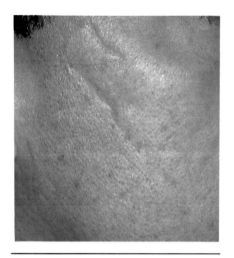

Surgical scar before laser treatment.

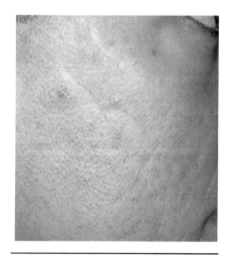

After four laser treatments.

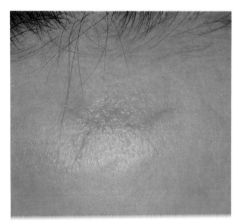

Forehead scar before laser treatment.

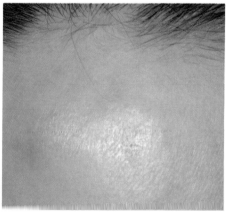

After one laser treatment.

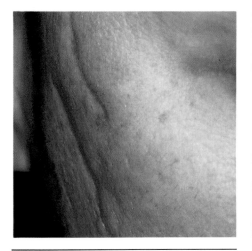

Surgical scar before laser treatment.

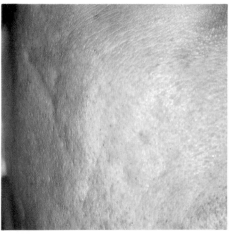

After four laser treatments. Notice depressed scar has almost completely risen to level of rest of skin due to new collagen formation. Further laser treatments needed to completely resolve the remaining scar.

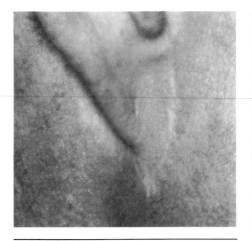

White scar before laser treatment.

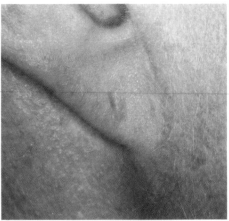

After one laser treatment.

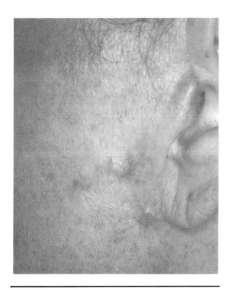

Thickened scar before laser treatment.

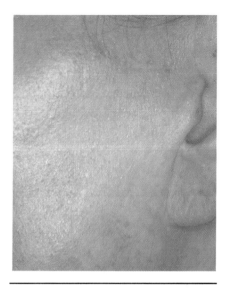

After six laser treatments.

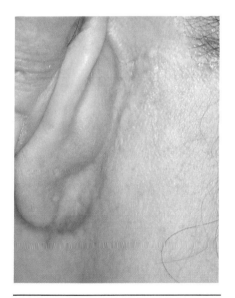

Thickened, red scar following facelift surgery before laser treatment.

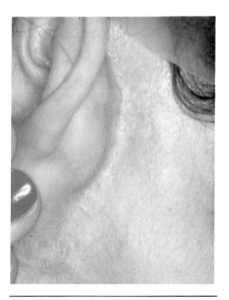

After one laser treatment.

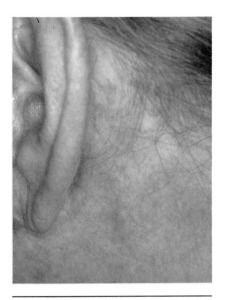

Red scar following facelift surgery before laser treatment.

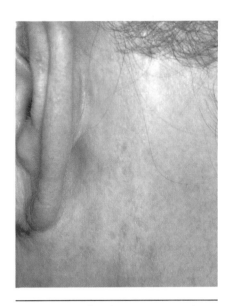

Removal of redness exposed white scar present underneath the redness.

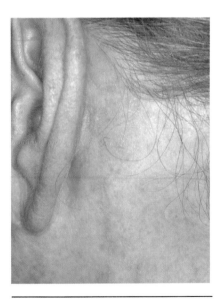

White scar after two laser treatments.

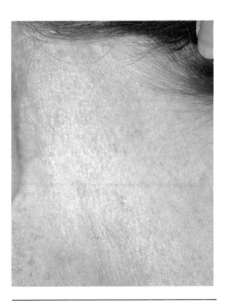

White scar after eight laser treatments. Notice skin has returned to its normal color and texture.

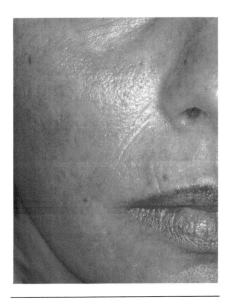

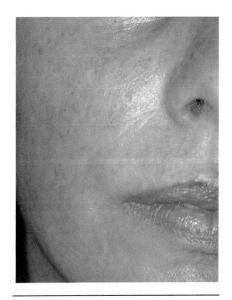

Surgical scar on the upper lip, smile line wrinkles, broken capillaries and sun-damaged skin before laser treatment.

After two and one laser treatments, respectively. Notice the rejuvenating effect on the texture of the sun-damaged skin.

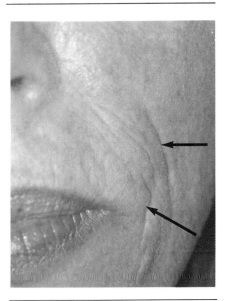

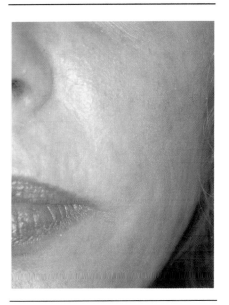

Two surgical scars (indicated by arrows), broken capillaries and sun-damaged skin before laser treatment.

After six and one laser treatments, respectively. Notice the rejuvenating and smoothing effect on the skin.

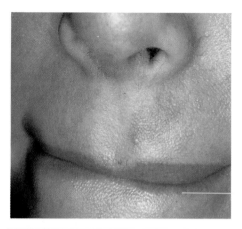

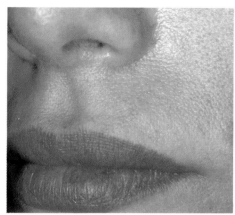

Redness resulting from injury to the upper lip.

After one laser treatment.

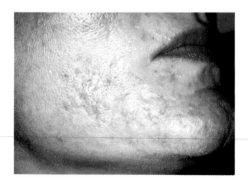

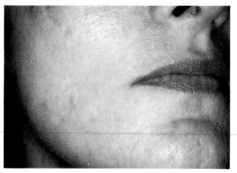

Scarring from rare condition called systemic lupus, before laser treatment. This condition is caused by loss of collagen. Acne scarring is also caused by loss of collagen due to the inflammation in skin associated with acne.

After four laser treatments.

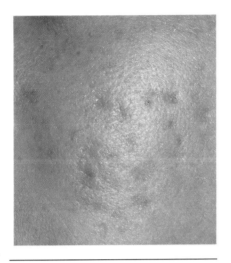

Acne scarring before laser treatment.

After one laser treatment.

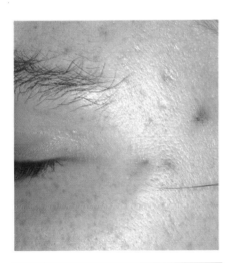

Acne scarring before laser treatment.

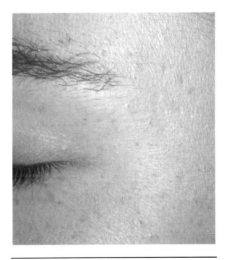

After two laser treatments.

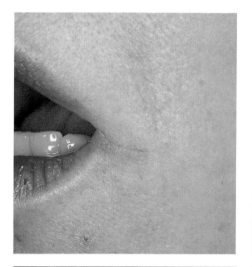

Red facial scar before laser treatment.

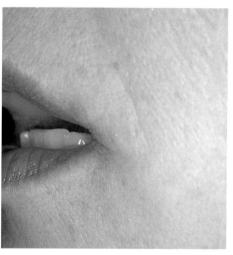

After one laser treatment.

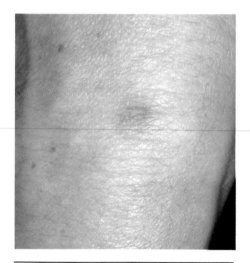

Red scar following injury before laser treatment.

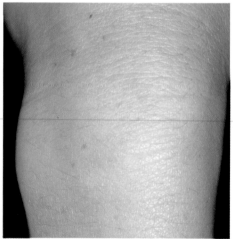

After two laser treatments.

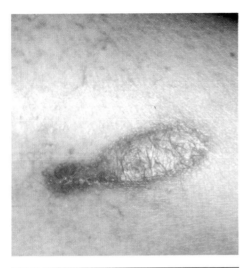

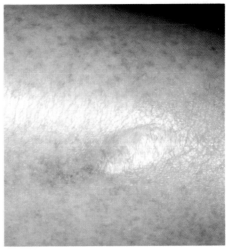

Scar resulting from a complication of sclerotherapy, before laser treatment.

After two laser treatments.

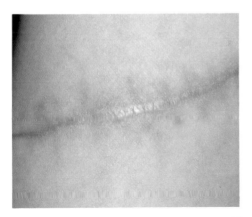

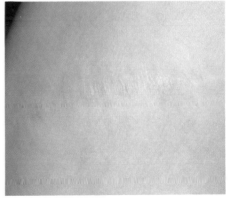

Red surgical scar before laser treatment.

After two laser treatments.

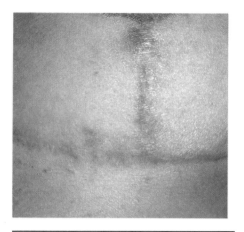

Scar following breast reduction surgery before laser treatment.

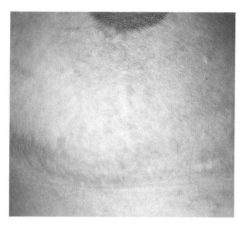

After one laser treatment.

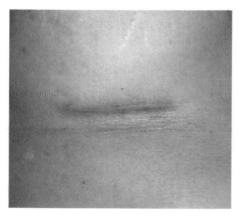

Thickened, red scar following breast implant surgery before laser treatment.

After three laser treatments.

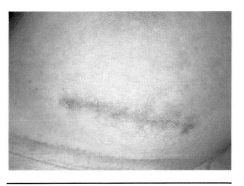

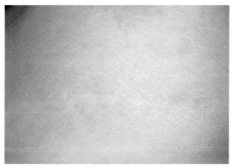

Flat, red scar following breast implant surgery before laser treatment.

After two laser treatments.

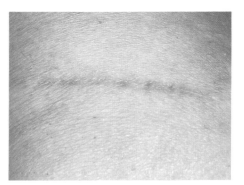

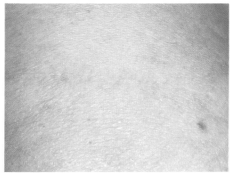

Red depressed scar following orthopedic surgery to the knee before laser treatment.

After two laser treatments.

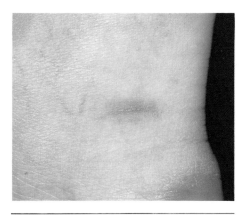 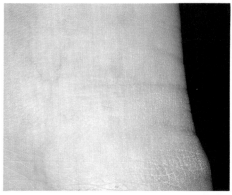

Scar following liposuction before laser treatment.

After one laser treatment.

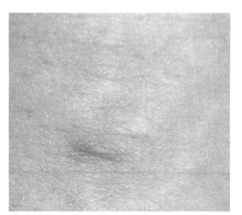 

Scar following liposuction before treatment.

After one laser treatment.

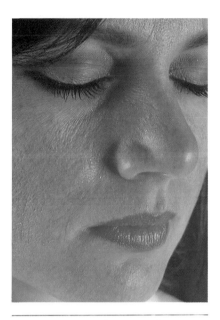

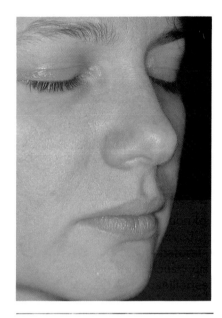

My own face after sun damage sustained during my childhood in Australia before laser treatment.

After two laser treatments. Notice the texture of skin has been rejuvenated. In addition to the capillaries being removed, my nose returned to its natural shape after it was previously distended by the excess capillaries.

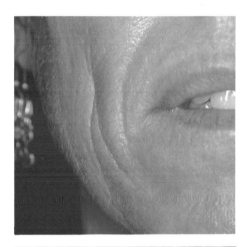

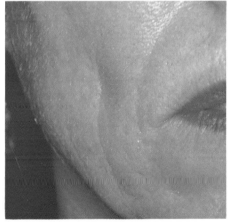

Capillaries and premature, deep wrinkles due to sun damage and the effects of time before laser treatment.

Rejuvenated skin after two laser treatments.

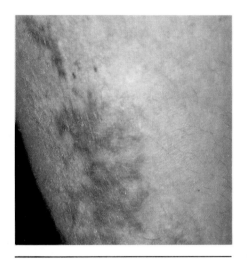

Scar from rare liposuction complication before laser treatment.

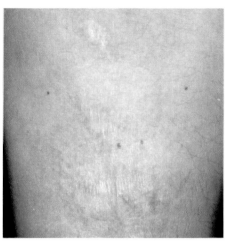

After one laser treatment.

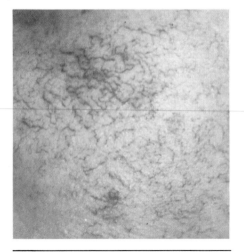

Severe broken capillaries before
laser treatment.

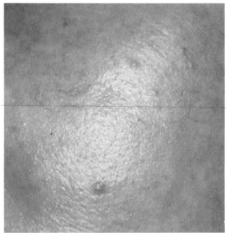

After six laser treatments.

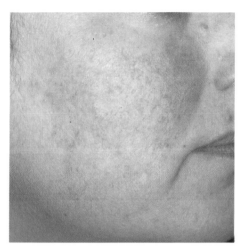

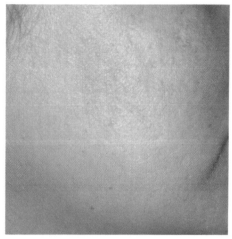

Broken capillaries due to acne rosacea before laser treatment.

After one laser treatment.

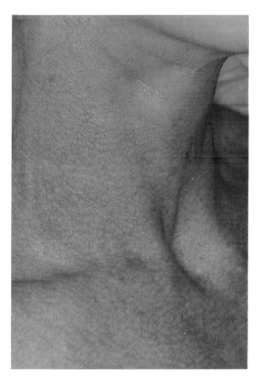

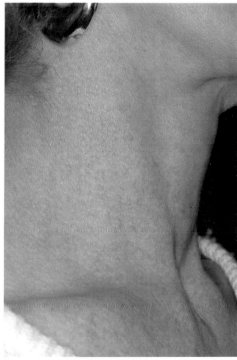

Redness on the neck and chest due to severe sun damage before laser treatment.

After one laser treatment.

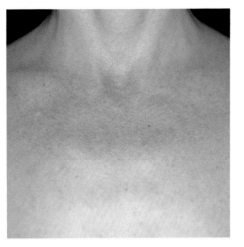

Redness due to moderate sun damage on the chest before laser treatment.

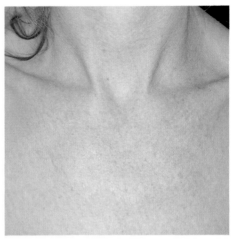

After one laser treatment.

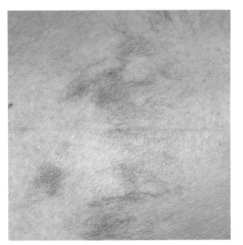

Red, telangiectatic matting, a rare complication of sclerotherapy before treatment.

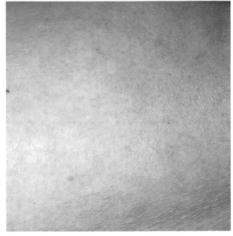

After four further sclerotherapy treatments.

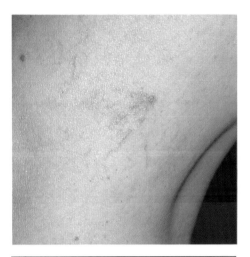

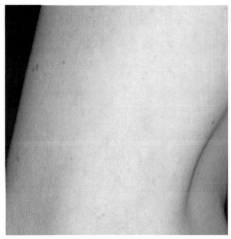

Spider veins before treatment.

After sclerotherapy.

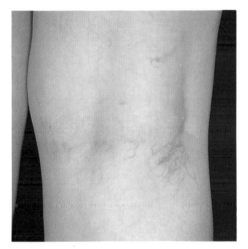

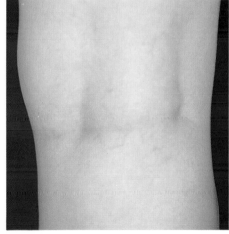

Varicosities and spider veins before treatment.

After sclerotherapy.

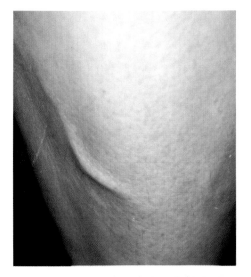 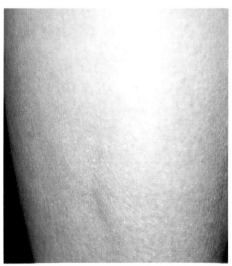

Varicose vein before treatment. | After sclerotherapy.

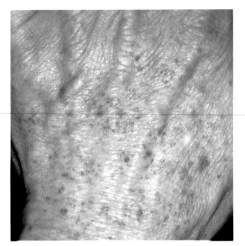 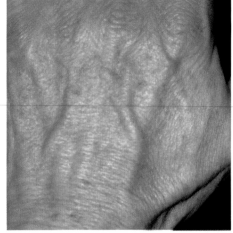

Sun age spots on back of the hand before laser treatment. | After one laser treatment.

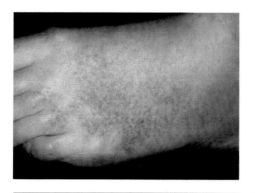

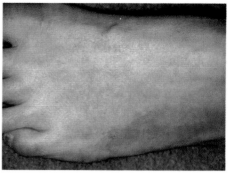

Excessive broken capillaries before laser treatment.

After two laser treatments.

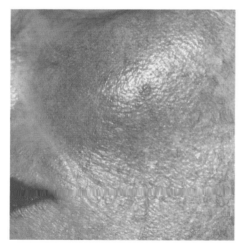

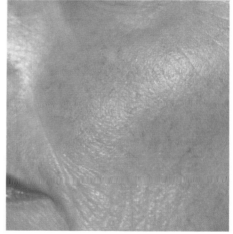

Broken capillaries due to severe sun damage before laser treatment.

After one laser treatment.

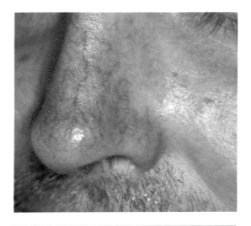

Red nose due to excess broken capillaries before laser treatment.

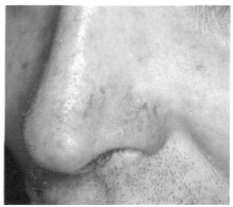

After six laser treatments.

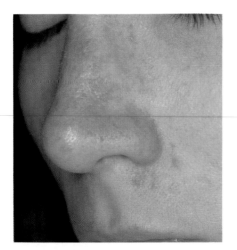

Red nose due to excess broken capillaries before laser treatment.

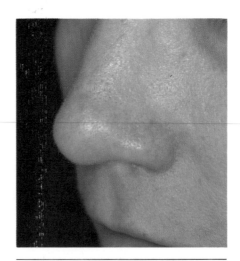

After two laser treatments.

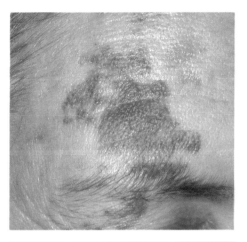

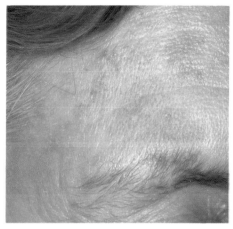

Portwine birthmark before laser treatment.

After eight laser treatments.

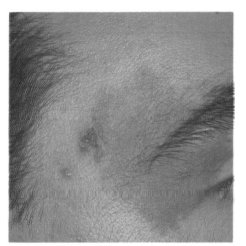

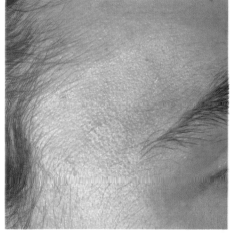

Portwine birthmark before laser treatment.

After three laser treatments.

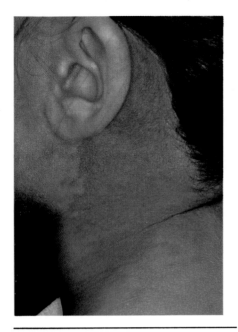

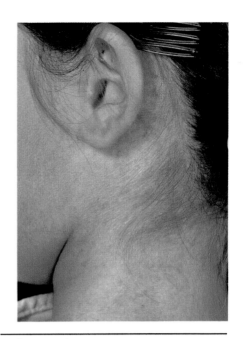

Portwine birthmark before laser treatment.

After two laser treatments.

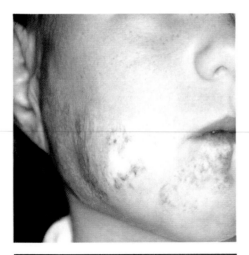

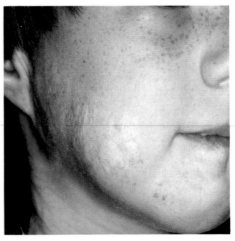

Cavernous hemangioma before laser treatment.

After three laser treatments. Notice skin has also repigmented in lower cheek area.

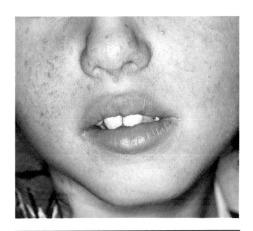

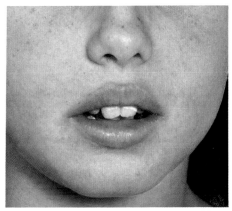

Tuberous sclerosis before laser treatment.

After one laser treatment.

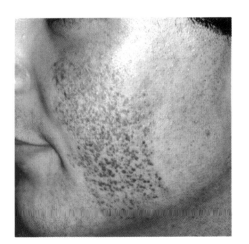

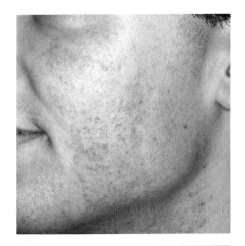

Benign brown birthmark (nevus spillus) before laser treatment.

After two laser treatments.

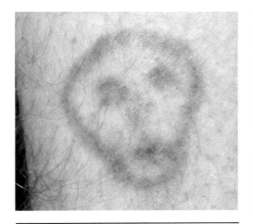

Non-professional tattoo before laser treatment.

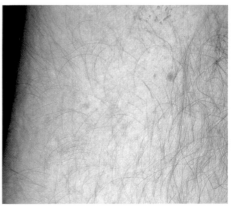

After four laser treatments.

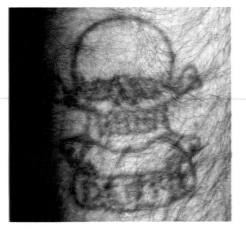

Professional tattoo before laser treatment.

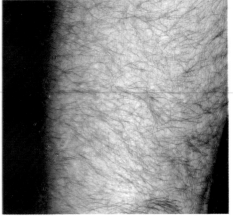

After eight laser treatments.

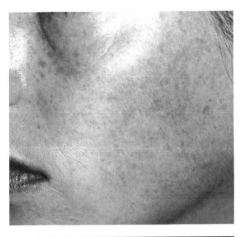 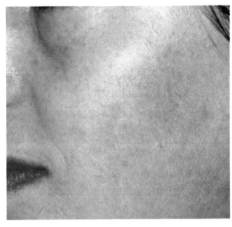

Excessive freckling due to sun damage.

After trichloroacetic acid (TCA) peel.

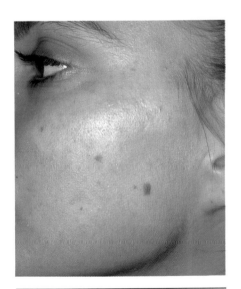 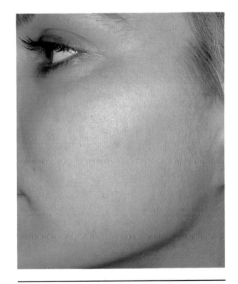

Broken capillaries and pigmentation due to sun damage before treatment.

After one laser treatment and trichloroacetic acid (TCA) peel.

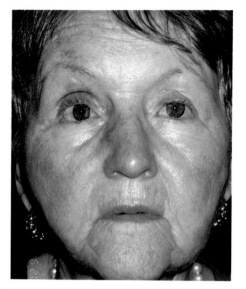

Before permanent make-up.

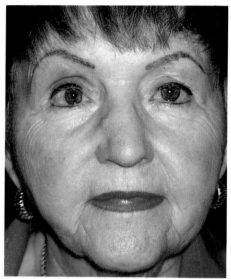

After eyebrow and eyelid enhance-ment.

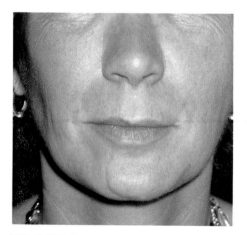

Before permanent make-up.

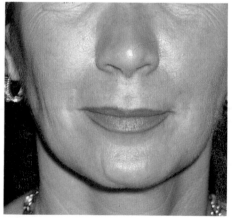

After lip enhancement.

Photographs on this page courtesy of Margot Schweifler, R.N.

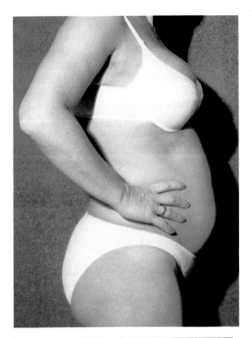

One month after delivery of a baby before using Ultratone™.

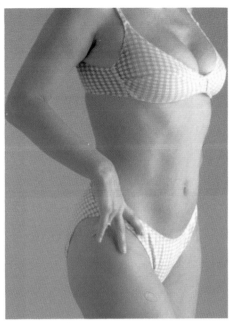

Three months after using Ultratone™ without additional exercise.

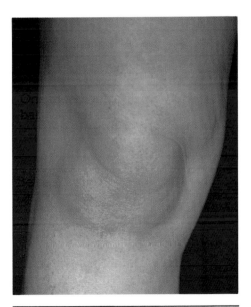

Before Ultratone™.

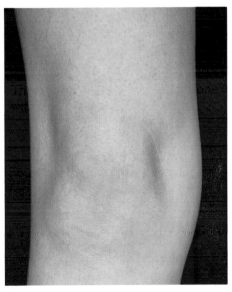

Four month after using Ultratone™ (approximately 30 sessions).

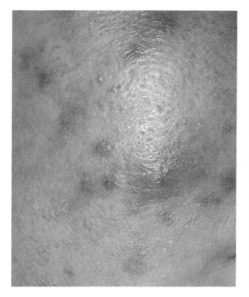

Complication of dermabrasion and chemical peels before laser treatment.

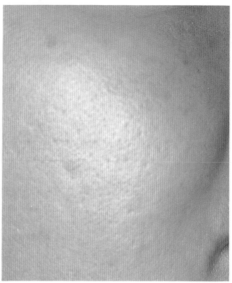

After two laser treatments.

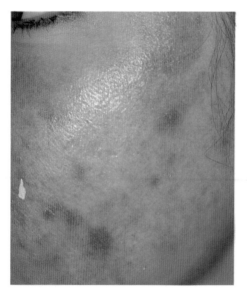

Complication of dermabrasion and chemical peels before laser treatment.

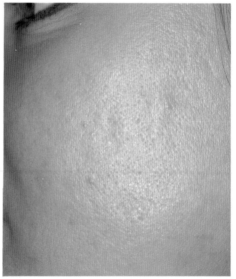

After two laser treatments.

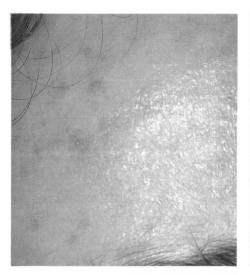

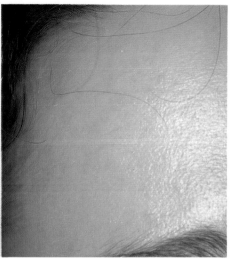

Complication of dermabrasion and chemical peels before laser treatment.

After two laser treatments.

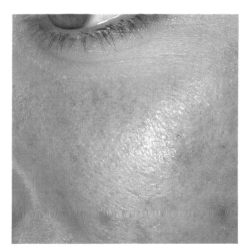

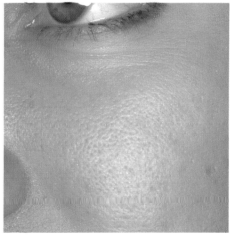

Complication of dermabrasion and chemical peels before laser treatment.

After two laser treatments.

AFTERWORD

WHY HAVE COSMETIC SURGERY?

Having read through all this, you are probably wondering why anyone would want to have cosmetic surgery at all. Don't forget that although the list of complications is long, they do not always occur and even if they do, most resolve without long-term problems. Some complications can also be avoided by being aware of them before surgery, and by meticulous attention to post-operative care. However, this does not mean that cosmetic surgery should be taken lightly. You should always be aware that nothing in medicine can be guaranteed, because it is impossible to accurately predict exactly how every individual will react to a particular procedure or how well they will heal.

Choosing your doctor well is also important. While in the next few years we can expect further advances, cosmetic surgery is certainly here to stay and can provide very beneficial results for many people.

The fact is, that the end results make the overwhelming majority of people who have cosmetic surgery happier than they were before. Long after the swelling and discomfort are forgotten, a younger face looks back from the mirror to face the world every day.

In conclusion, I hope this book has given you a better understanding of how to take care of your skin, as well as giving you a better insight into the world of cosmetic treatments and surgery.

My sincere hope is that whatever you decide to do, it will be a choice you have made for yourself and not one based on someone else's opinion or society at large.

BIBLIOGRAPHY

Allen, James. *As A Man Thinketh.* Philadelphia: Running Press, 1989.

American Institute of Permanent Color Technology, The. 1-800-772-4728.

Beck, Aaron T. *Love is Never Enough.* New York: Penguin Books, 1988.

Bonus, Nancy. *Food Without Fear.* California: Hi-Tech Graphics and Printing, 1992.

Branden, Nathaniel. *The Psychology of Self-Esteem.* New York: Bantam Books, 1987.

Burns, David D. *Feeling Good.* New York: New American Library, 1981.

Campbell, Eileen. *A Dancing Star.* London: The Aquarian Press, 1991.

Collins, Gary Max and Stephen C. Paul. *Illuminations.* San Francisco: Harper, 1991.

Course in Miracles, A. Glen Ellen, CA: Foundation for Inner Peace, 1976.

Davis, Wynn. *The Best of Success.* Illinois: Quotations Publishing Company, 1988.

Eichenbaum, Louise and Susie Orbach. *What do Women Want.* New York: Coward-McCann Inc., 1984.

Ellis, Albert and Robert A. Harper. *A New Guide to Rational Living.* Wilshire Book Company, 1975.

Ford, Edward. *Choosing to Love.* Arizona: Harper & Row, 1983.

Fox, Emmet. *Life After Death.* Marina Del Rey, CA: De Vorss & Co, 1966.

Fox, Emmet. *The Sermon on the Mount.* San Francisco: Harper Collins, 1964.

Gendlin, Eugene T. *Focusing.* New York: Bantam Books, 1988.

Gibran, Kahlil. *The Prophet.* New York: Alfred A. Knopf, 1971.

Goldsmith, Joel S. *The Art of Spiritual Healing.* San Francisco: Harper Collins, 1959.

Gray, John. *What You Feel, You Can Heal.* Mill Valley, CA: Heart Publishing, 1984.

Hayward, Susan. *You Have A Purpose/ Begin it Now.* Avalon, Australia: In-Tune Books, 1991.

Hill, Napoleon. *Think and Grow Rich.* Conneticutt: Fawcett World Library, 1960.

Holland, Jack H. *Man's Victorious Spirit.* Monterey, CA: Hudson-Cohan Publishing Company, 1971.

Holmes, Ernest. *Creative Ideas.* ed.,comp., Willis Kinnear. Los Angeles: Science of Mind Communications, 1973.

Holmes, Ernest. *The Science of Mind.* New York: G.P. Putnam's Sons, 1988.

Horney, Karen. *Self-Analysis.* New York: W. W. Norton and Co., 1942.

Horney, Karen. *The Neurotic Personality of Our Time.* New York: W.W. Norton and Co., 1941.

Hutchison, Michael. *MegaBrain.* New York: Ballantine Books, 1991.

Maltz, Maxwell. *Psycho-Cybernetics and Self-Fulfillment.* New York: Bantam Books, 1970.

Miller, Alice. *Thou Shalt Not Be Aware.* New York: New American Library, 1986.

New, Richard. *Vibrational Medicine.* Santa Fe: Gerber, Bear and Company, 1988.

Powell, John. *Fully Human, Fully Alive.* Texas: Argus Communications, 1976.

Powell, John. *Why Am I Afraid to Love?*
Texas: Argus Communications, 1967.

Powell, John. *Why Am I Afraid to Tell You
Who I Am?* Texas: Argus Communications,
1969.

Predeteanu, Constantin. *The ABC's of
Cosmetics.* Brookfield Hills, MI: Institute
Predete Publishing Company, 1987.

Puryear, Herbert B. *The Edgar Cayce Primer.*
New York: Bantam Books, 1982.

Roman, Sanaya. *Personal Power Through
Awareness.* Tiburon, CA: H.J. Kramer Inc.,
1986.

Scheibner, Adrianna. *How To Look Young
Longer.* Australia: Simon & Schuster, 1991.

Spalding, Baird T. *The Life and Teaching of
the Masters of the Far East.* Vol.4. Marina Del
Rey, CA: De Vorss and Company, 1976.

The Living Bible. Wheaton, Illinois: Tyndale
House Publishers, Inc., 1971.

Viscott, David. *Risking.* New York: Pocket
Books, 1977.

Viscott, David. *The Language of Feeling.*
New York: Pocket Books, 1977.

Winter, Ruth. *Consumers Dictionary of
Cosmetic Ingredients.* New York: Crown
Publishers, 1989.

Yogananda, Paramahansa. *The Essence of
Self-Realization.* California: Crystal Clarity
Publishers, 1991.

Yogananda, Paramahansa, int. *The Sermon
on The Mount.* Dallas: Amrita Foundation,
1979.

Yogananda, Paramahansa. *The Law of
Success.* Los Angeles: Self-Realization
Fellowship, 1990.

INDEX

ORDER FORM

☐ **Yes,** please send me a complimentary *The Essence of Beauty* Hemisphonic Tape.
    ☐ Easy Listening.   ☐ Pastoral Harmonies.
    ☐ Classical.   ☐ Tropical Ocean.

☐ **Yes,** I would like extra copies of *The Essence of Beauty*
    ☐ Hard Cover @ $29.95 plus shipping and handling.
    ☐ Soft Cover @ $16.95 plus shipping and handling.

☐ **Yes,** I would like more information on the **Amber Essence Skin Care** line.

☐ **Yes,** I would like to receive the quarterly magazine *The Essence of Health and Beauty.*

Name _____

Address _____

City _____ State _____ Zip _____

Payment: ☐ Check ☐ Visa ☐ MasterCard ☐ Amex
Make checks payable to: **A&A PUBLISHERS & DISTRIBUTORS**

Card Number _____ Expiration Date _____

Name on Card _____ Signature _____

ITEM DESCRIPTION	QUANTITY	COST
SUB-TOTAL		
SALES TAX: (Please add 8.25% for books shipped to California)........		
SHIPPING: (Book rate: $3.00 for the first book and 75¢ for each additional book. Surface shipping may take 3-4 weeks)		
TOTAL:		

Telephone orders call Toll Free **(800) 262-3720**
Fax orders **(805) 640-1216**
or fill out this order form and mail to:
A&A Publishers & Distributors
410 Bryant Circle, Suite H, Ojai, CA 93023